Companion Guide to Measurement and Evaluation for Kinesiology

Companion Guide to Measurement and Evaluation for Kinesiology

David Tomchuk, MS, ATC, LAT, CSCS
Missouri Valley College

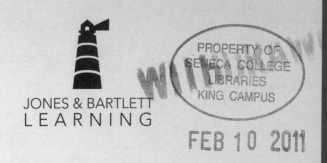

JONES & BARTLETT
LEARNING

World Headquarters
Jones & Bartlett Learning
40 Tall Pine Drive
Sudbury, MA 01776
978-443-5000
info@jblearning.com
www.jblearning.com

Jones & Bartlett Learning
Canada
6339 Ormindale Way
Mississauga, Ontario L5V 1J2
Canada

Jones & Bartlett Learning
International
Barb House, Barb Mews
London W6 7PA
United Kingdom

Jones & Bartlett Learning books and products are available through most bookstores and online booksellers. To contact Jones & Bartlett Learning directly, call 800-832-0034, fax 978-443-8000, or visit our website, www.jblearning.com.

Substantial discounts on bulk quantities of Jones & Bartlett Learning publications are available to corporations, professional associations, and other qualified organizations. For details and specific discount information, contact the special sales department at Jones & Bartlett Learning via the above contact information or send an email to specialsales@jblearning.com.

The author, editor, and publisher have made every effort to provide accurate information. However, they are not responsible for errors, omissions, or for any outcomes related to the use of the contents of this book and take no responsibility for the use of the products and procedures described. Treatments and side effects described in this book may not be applicable to all people; likewise, some people may require a dose or experience a side effect that is not described herein. Drugs and medical devices are discussed that may have limited availability controlled by the Food and Drug Administration (FDA) for use only in a research study or clinical trial. Research, clinical practice, and government regulations often change the accepted standard in this field. When consideration is being given to use of any drug in the clinical setting, the health care provider or reader is responsible for determining FDA status of the drug, reading the package insert, and reviewing prescribing information for the most up-to-date recommendations on dose, precautions, and contraindications, and determining the appropriate usage for the product. This is especially important in the case of drugs that are new or seldom used.

Production Credits

Publisher, Higher Education: Cathleen Sether
Senior Acquisitions Editor: Shoshanna Goldberg
Senior Associate Editor: Amy L. Bloom
Senior Editorial Assistant: Kyle Hoover
Production Manager: Julie Champagne Bolduc
Production Editor: Jessica Steele Newfell
Associate Marketing Manager: Jody Sullivan
V.P., Manufacturing and Inventory Control:
    Therese Connell

Composition: Cape Cod Compositors, Inc.
Cover Design: Scott Moden
Assistant Photo Researcher: Rebecca Ritter
Cover Image: © ImageryMajestic/ShutterStock, Inc.
Photo Credits: (p. 83) © Robert J. Daveant/ShutterStock,
    Inc., (p. 110) © Mark Herreid/Dreamstime.com
Printing and Binding: Malloy, Inc.
Cover Printing: Malloy, Inc.

Library of Congress Cataloging-in-Publication Data
Tomchuk, David.
    Companion guide to measurement and evaluation for kinesiology / David Tomchuk.
        p.   cm.
    Includes bibliographical references and index.
    ISBN 978-0-7637-7610-7 (pbk. : alk. paper)
    1. Physical fitness—Testing.   2. Kinesiology.   I. Title.
    GV436.T66 2011
    613.7—dc22

                                                                        2010022244

6048

Printed in the United States of America
14 13 12 11 10   10 9 8 7 6 5 4 3 2 1

Contents

Preface   ix
Acknowledgments   xi

Chapter 1   **Introduction to Timing and Fitness Test Batteries**   1
             Fitnessgram®/Activitygram®   3
             YMCA Physical Fitness Test   4
             ACSM Fitness Test   4
             President's Challenge Fitness Test   5
             Functional Fitness Test for Community-Residing Older Adults   5
             NFL (American Football) Test Battery   6

Chapter 2   **Body Composition**   7
             Chest/Pectoral Skinfold Site   8
             Subscapular Skinfold Site   9
             Midaxillary Skinfold Site   10
             Suprailiac Skinfold Site   11
             Abdominal Skinfold Site   12
             Triceps Skinfold Site   12
             Biceps Skinfold Site   14
             Thigh Skinfold Site   15
             Calf Skinfold Site   16
             Body Mass Index (BMI)   16
             Waist-to-Hip Ratio (WHR)   19

Chapter 3   **Flexibility Testing**   **23**
                  Sit-and-Reach Test   24
                  Modified Sit-and-Reach Test   26
                  YMCA Sit-and-Reach Test   28
                  Sit-and-Reach Wall Test   29
                  V-Sit-and-Reach Test   30
                  Back-Saver Sit-and-Reach Test   32
                  Modified Back-Saver Sit-and-Reach Test   34
                  Chair Sit-and-Reach Test   35
                  Trunk Lift Test   37
                  Trunk-and-Neck Extension Test   39
                  Shoulder Lift Test   40
                  Shoulder-and-Wrist Elevation Test   42
                  Back Scratch Test   43

Chapter 4   **Local Muscular Endurance Testing**   **47**
                  YMCA Bench Press Test   48
                  NFL-225 Bench Press Test   50
                  Pull-Ups for Endurance Test   52
                  Modified Pull-Ups for Endurance Test   54
                  Flexed Arm-Hang Test   56
                  Dips for Endurance Test   57
                  Push-Ups for Endurance Test   59
                  Modified Push-Ups for Endurance Test   61
                  Arm-Curl Test   63
                  Sit-Ups for Endurance Test   65
                  Abdominal Curl for Endurance Test   68
                  Static Leg Endurance Test   69
                  30-Second Chair Stand Test   71
                  Back Extensor Endurance Test   73

Chapter 5   **Balance Testing**   **75**
                  Stork Stand Test   76
                  Bass Stick Test (Lengthwise)   78
                  Bass Stick Test (Crosswise)   79
                  Tandem Stance Test   81
                  Balance Beam Walk Test   82
                  Tandem Walking Test   84
                  Timed 360° Turn Test   85
                  Modified Bass Dynamic Balance Test   87
                  Modified Sideward Leap Test   89
                  Star Excursion Balance Test (SEBT)   90

Chapter 6   **Strength Testing**   **93**

Handgrip Strength (Dynamometer) Test   94
1-Repetition Maximum (1RM) Bench Press Test   96
1-Repetition Maximum (1RM) Squat Test   98
Sit-Ups for Strength Test   100
Adbominal Stage Test   101
Pull-Ups for Strength Test   104
Dips for Strength Test   106

Chapter 7   **Power Testing**   **109**

Standing Broad Jump Test   110
Sargent's Test   112
Vane-Slat Apparatus Method   114
1-Leg Hop Test   116
3-Hop Test   118
5-Jump Test   120
Crossover Hop Test   121
6-Meter Timed Hop Test   123
Square Hop Test   124
Side Hop Test   126
Hop and Stop Test   127
Seated Medicine Ball Throw Test   131
Seated Shot Put Test   133
Standing Medicine Ball Chest Pass Test   135
Standing Medicine Ball Throw Test   137
Backward Overhead Medicine Ball Throw Test   139

Chapter 8   **Aerobic Capacity and Cardiorespiratory Fitness Testing**   **141**

Cooper Test: 9-Minute or 12-Minute Walk/Run Test   142
1-Mile (1.6-Kilometer) or 1.5-Mile (2.4-Kilometer) Run/Walk Test   144
Submaximal Mile (1.6-Kilometer) Track Jog Test   146
1-Mile (1.6-Kilometer) Walk Test   147
Rockport 1-Mile (1.6-Kilometer) Fitness Walking Test   148
3-Mile (4.8-Kilometer) Walk Test   150
6-Minute Walk Test   150
2-Minute Step-in-Place Test   153
YMCA 3-Minute Step Test   154
Queens College Step Test   155
Harvard Step Test   157
Harvard Step Test for Junior and Senior High Males   158
Harvard Step Test for Junior High, Senior High, and College Females   161
Harvard Step Test for Elementary School-Aged Males and Females   162
Hoosier Endurance Shuttle Run Test   164
Progressive Aerobic Cardiovascular Endurance Run (PACER) Test   165

	Continuous Multistage Fitness (MFT) Test	167
	Yo-Yo Endurance (Continuous) Test	169
	Yo-Yo Intermittent Endurance (YYIE) Test	171
	Yo-Yo Intermittent Recovery (YYIR) Test	173
Chapter 9	**Anaerobic Capacity (Anaerobic Power) Testing**	**177**
	60-Yard (54.8-Meter) Shuttle Test	178
	300-Yard (274-Meter) Shuttle Test	179
	Line Drill Test	180
	Triple 120-Meter (131-Yard) Shuttle Test	183
	40-Meter Maximal Shuttle Run (40-M MST) Test	185
	Repeated Shuttle Sprint Ability (RSSA) Test	186
	Repeated 220-Yard (201-Meter) Sprint Test	188
	5-Meter (5.5-Yard) Multiple Shuttle Test	190
Chapter 10	**Agility Testing**	**193**
	Right Boomerang Run Test	194
	Sidestepping Test	196
	Edgren Side Step Test	197
	SEMO Agility Test	198
	AAHPERD Shuttle Run Test	200
	Barrow Zigzag Run Test	202
	T-Test	203
	Illinois Agility Test	205
	Up and Back (UAB) Agility Test	207
	505 Agility Test	209
	Pro-Agility Test	210
	3-Cone Drill	212
	Nebraska Agility Run Test	214
	4-Corner Shuttle Run Test	215
	Balsom (Soccer) Agility Test	217
	Hexagon Test	219
	8-Feet Up-and-Go Test	221
Chapter 11	**Speed, Speed Endurance, and Acceleration Testing**	**223**
	40-Yard (37-Meter) Sprint (Dash) Test	224
	Kalamen 50-Yard (45.5-Meter) Test	226
	40-Yard (36.5-Meter) Repeated Sprint Test	227
	Bangsbo Sprint Test	229
	10-Meter (10.9-Yard) Triangle Sprint Test	230
Index		**233**

Preface

There are a variety of textbooks to choose from when planning and teaching a measurement and evaluation course. These textbooks typically consist of a limited number of physical fitness tests interspersed between information on statistical analysis methodology. A fitness test that is not properly set up and administered will give an incorrect or unreliable score, inevitably leading to inaccurate results.

Companion Guide to Measurement and Evaluation for Kinesiology is intended to be a simple measurement and evaluation textbook that is a "how-to" reference and a practical resource for use in both the classroom and the professional world. For each test, the book gives the objective, age range, appropriateness, necessary equipment, required personnel, set-up instructions, scoring instructions, and a checklist to ensure proper administration. The book covers many different physical fitness tests and test batteries rather than the statistical analysis methods and methodologies found in most measurement and evaluation texts.

This book is intended to be a supplemental textbook in measurement and evaluation courses that can be adapted to many different health-related academic majors. It will be useful for students in the fields of athletic training, physical education, exercise science, kinesiology, exercise physiology, and strength and conditioning, and it will be a handy resource for any health-related fitness professionals. This book may also be valuable to health-related majors who change employment settings or positions within their field and need to refresh their skills or learn how to perform physical fitness tests for different populations.

While this book includes some common physical fitness test batteries, including a brief description of the target populations, recent graduates do not need to rely solely on prefabricated fitness test batteries. My hope is that they will utilize their understanding of the measurement and evaluation process and their knowledge of the human body to create physical fitness test batteries that will properly measure the specific populations with which they are working.

All of the physical fitness tests described in this book are field tests that are easy and inexpensive to administer. Most of the tests require nothing more technical than a stopwatch, a tape measure, an open area, and some cones. Additionally, many of the fitness tests do not require an additional test assistant. High-quality photographs and figures show the proper set up and administration of each physical fitness test. Accurate photographs and figures illustrating important points and procedures attempt to limit potential measurement errors.

Whether you use this book to add a new physical fitness test to your current test battery, to create a new test of your own, to utilize an already created test battery, or to keep as a reference, I hope you find *Companion Guide to Measurement and Evaluation for Kinesiology* a valuable resource.

The clipboard icon represents the place where the test administrator should stand during the test.

The whistle icon shows where the test assistant (or assistants) should stand during the test.

Finally, the running shoes icon represents the path of the performer who is completing the test.

Additionally, the illustrations in this text are shaded to represent the speed at which the test performer must move.

The light footprints represent the segments of the test during which the performer should be moving at a slower pace by walking or jogging.

Similarly, the dark footprints represent the parts of the test during which the performer should be moving at a faster pace by running or sprinting.

Finally, the test performer should always be moving in the direction of the footprints and the arrows as depicted by the illustrations.

■ NOTES ON THIS TEXT

A practical resource for both students and professionals, *Companion Guide to Measurement and Evaluation for Kinesiology* includes photographs and illustrations that depict a variety of physical fitness tests and test batteries. In order to represent the speed, direction, and placement necessary for each test, the illustrations in this text include three different icons: a clipboard, a whistle, and a pair of running shoes.

Acknowledgments

First, I would like to thank the Missouri Valley College library staff of Pam Reeder, Sheeba Love, and Mary Slater. They were instrumental in finding articles and additional references that strengthened this book.

Thank you to Kylee Hawes, Jami Mayberry, Julie McNabb, Rachel Pike, Josh Lammert, Alex Thompson, Andre Taylor, Jennifer Asberry, and Abbey Humphrey, who allowed themselves to be photographed and drawn for this work and who provided research and organizational assistance.

I also would like to thank David A. Robertson, MA, ABD, for his careful review of the text.

Finally, thank you to Jami Mayberry and Julie McNabb for their initial drawings, which were the basis for the artwork in this textbook, which makes this textbook special and unique.

Introduction to Timing and Fitness Test Batteries

■ TIMING

Establishing an accurate time is crucial for any fitness test, particularly tests of agility, speed, speed endurance, or acceleration. Accuracy may be achieved by utilizing a stopwatch (hand timing) or an electronic timing system (electronic timing).

Hand timing can result in many potential measurement errors. An improperly or poorly trained timer can mistakenly give a test performer an inflated or deflated time. Even an experienced timer may have a predisposition in favor or against the test performer, which may result in an inflated or deflated time. A delay in initiating and/or stopping the stopwatch cannot be fully prevented, but it may be controlled and limited. Several solutions to the potential sources of hand timing measurement errors are discussed as follows.

An individual who is not experienced with using a stopwatch should not be the sole timer.

This person should be paired with an experienced timer or practice their timing skills against an electronic timing system. All timers should use the index finger to start and stop the stopwatch. The thumb should not be utilized, as it has a slower reaction time than the index finger.

It is difficult to determine if bias is occurring. There are two possible solutions: having a second experienced individual timing the trial or utilizing electronic timing. These solutions are not always practical, however. If a test administrator believes bias is occurring, the test administrator should personally time the performer.

The natural delay in initiating and/or stopping the stopwatch is a common source of timing errors. Such errors may occur at either the initiation or the conclusion of the trial. Initially, errors are the result of the natural delay between when the test performer is told to begin (or initiates) the trial and when the test administrator reacts and begins timing the trial. At the conclusion of the trial, there is a natural delay between the time when the test performer crosses the finish line and when the test administrator reacts to stop timing. Additionally, the timer's anticipation of when the test performer will cross the finish line may differ from when the test performer actually crosses the finish line.

To control these reaction-time delays, properly trained and experienced timers should be utilized. Both errors described above still occur with experienced timers. To minimize these errors, the timer should be the individual who initiates the test performer's beginning of the trial. This solution is practical only for tests that are initiated from and conclude at the same location.

When the timer and test performer begin a trial at different locations, a test assistant should be placed at the starting line to initiate the trial. The test assistant will raise his or her arm while verbally giving the test performer the "set" command and drop the arm rapidly when the verbal "go" command is given to the test performer. This function also may be performed by using a starting gun or similar apparatus. Proper communication between the timer and the test assistant is essential to proper initiation of the time.

If a test assistant is not available to start the test performer's trial and the trial will begin and conclude at different locations, the timer may choose to begin timing the trial on the test performer's first movement. This process, however, provides a distinct advantage to the test performer because the timer loses additional control initiating the time, possibly resulting in additional inaccuracies.

At the finish line, the timer must anticipate when the test performer will cross the finish line and coordinate stopping the time at that exact moment. The best way to control this timing error is if the test performer does not

decelerate before crossing the finish line. The test administrator should encourage the test performer to "run through" the finish line and not decelerate during the final strides of the trial to ensure proper timing.

Electronic timing systems are considered the gold standard and are generally reported, unless indicated otherwise. Electronic timing systems are becoming more cost effective to purchase and simpler to set up. An electronic timing system should be utilized whenever possible and practical.

Hand times should be converted to electronic times to be properly recorded and reported. As a general rule, if a timer utilizes a stopwatch properly (with the index finger), has no bias, and initiates and concludes the stopwatch properly, the resultant time will be 0.24 seconds *faster* than the same performance timed electronically. This is because of the delay in the timer initially starting the time, which leads to the hand time being artificially faster. To convert a hand time to an electronic time; *add* 0.24 seconds to the hand time result.

electronic time = hand time result + 0.24

■ TEST BATTERIES

A fitness test battery is a collection of separate fitness tests that are combined to evaluate an individual's physical fitness or athletic ability. Fitness test batteries can be either health related or skill related. The fitness test batteries presented in this section are ones that have been implemented by various fitness and athletic organizations. There are many fitness test batteries performed by many separate organizations. This section describes some common fitness test batteries. It is recommended that all test performers undergo and pass a physical examination before participating in any fitness tests or test batteries.

Health-related test batteries typically include tests that measure cardiorespiratory fitness, muscular strength, local muscular endurance, flexibility, and body composition. These tests are geared toward evaluating an individual's ability to perform the activities of daily life and leisurely physical activities, general fitness, and ability to lead an overall healthy life.

Skill-related test batteries typically include tests that measure cardiorespiratory fitness, local muscular endurance, muscular strength, flexibility, and body composition. However, skill-related test batteries usually also measure agility, speed, balance, and power of the test performers. These test batteries are performed to evaluate athletic talent. Each athletic activity emphasizes different criteria for success (performing well).

Whether using a fitness test battery that is presented in this textbook, one that is not, or one that has been created, it is imperative that the test administrator understands and properly implements the fitness test battery. Following the correct order of the individual fitness tests and the performance of those tests will ensure the most accurate score possible. The test administrator should also ensure that the test performers have adequate rest between test trials and individual tests that constitute the battery. Test administrators who create test batteries of their own should use their knowledge of the measurement and evaluation process and the human body to select physical fitness tests that properly measure the test population.

References are provided for the fitness test batteries described. Some organizations have forms and other documents that make recording of the fitness test battery easier.

■ FITNESSGRAM®/ACTIVITYGRAM®

Objective: Measure general fitness of children and young adults

Age Range: 5 to 17+

Test Components:

1. **Aerobic capacity**
   PACER (page 165) *or*
   1-mile run/walk test (page 144) *or*
   1-mile walk test (page 147)
2. **Body composition (K–12)**
   Sum of two skinfold measurements:
     Triceps (page 12)
     Medial calf (page 16)
   Alternative: Body mass index (BMI)
     (page 16)

3. **Abdominal strength and endurance**
   Curl-up test (page 68)
4. **Trunk extensor strength and flexibility**
   Trunk lift (page 37)
5. **Upper-body strength and endurance**
   Push-ups (page 59)
   Pull-ups (page 52)
   Modified pull-ups (page 54)
   Flexed arm-hang (page 56)
6. **Flexibility**
   Back-saver sit-and-reach test (page 32)
   Shoulder stretch (page 40)

References

Meredith, M. D., & Welk, C. J. (2007). *FITNESS GRAM®/ACTIVITYGRAM® test administration manual* (4th ed.). Champaign, IL: Human Kinetics.

Miller, D. K. (2006). *Measurement by the physical educator: Why and how* (5th ed.). New York: McGraw-Hill.

The Cooper Institute. http://www.cooperinstitute.org

■ YMCA PHYSICAL FITNESS TEST

Objective: Measure general fitness of adults

Age Range: 18 to 60+

Test Components:

1. **Body composition**
   Sum of four skinfold measurements:
   Abdomen (page 12)
   Suprailiac (page 11)
   Triceps (page 12)
   Thigh (page 15)
2. **Aerobic capacity**
   YMCA 3-minute step test (page 154)
   Bicycle ergometer (not described in this book)
3. **Flexibility**
   YMCA sit-and-reach test (page 28)
4. **Muscular strength**
   YMCA bench press test (page 48)
5. **Muscular endurance**
   YMCA half sit-up test (page 68)

References

Golding, L. A. (2000). *YMCA fitness testing and assessment manual* (4th ed.) Champaign, IL: Human Kinetics.

Miller, D. K. (2006). *Measurement by the physical educator: Why and how* (5th ed.). New York: McGraw-Hill.

■ ACSM FITNESS TEST

Objective: Measure general fitness of adults

Age Range: 20 to 60+

Test Components:

1. **Body composition**
   Body mass index (page 16)
   Waist-to-hip ratio (page 19)
2. **Flexibility**
   (YMCA) Sit-and-reach test (page 28)
3. **Muscular endurance**
   Male: Push-ups (page 59)
   Female: Modified push-ups (page 61)
4. **Aerobic capacity**
   Rockport 1-mile walking test (page 148)

References

American College of Sports Medicine. (2003). *ACSM's fitness book* (3rd ed.). Champaign, IL: Human Kinetics.

Miller, D. K. (2006). *Measurement by the physical educator: Why and how* (5th ed.). New York: McGraw-Hill.

■ PRESIDENT'S CHALLENGE FITNESS TEST

Objective: Measure general fitness of children

Age Range: 6 to 17

Test Components:

1. **Flexibility**
   V-sit-and-reach test (page 30)
2. **Muscular strength and endurance**
   Upper body
   Pull-ups (page 52) *or*
   (Right-angle) push-ups (same protocol as page 59, but the test performer lowers the body until a 90° angle at the elbows is created without lowering the chest to the mat, with one push-up being completed every 3 seconds) *or*
   Flexed-arm hang (page 56)

   Abdominal
   Curl-ups (page 68, with the test performer's arms in contact with the chest; the test performer's elbows should touch the thighs)
3. **Agility**
   Shuttle run test (page 215)
4. **Aerobic capacity**
   1-mile run/walk test (page 144; there are quarter- and half-mile variations for young children)

References

Miller, D. K. (2006). *Measurement by the physical educator: Why and how* (5th ed.). New York: McGraw-Hill.

The President's Challenge. http://www.presidents challenge.org

■ FUNCTIONAL FITNESS TEST FOR COMMUNITY-RESIDING OLDER ADULTS

Objective: Measure the physical and mobility abilities of independent senior citizens

Age Range: 60+

Test Components:

1. **Body composition**
   Body mass index (page 16)
2. **Flexibility**
   Upper body: Back scratch test (page 43)
   Lower body: Chair sit-and-reach test (page 35)
3. **Muscular strength and endurance**
   Upper body: Arm-curl test (page 63)
   Lower body: 30-second chair stand test (page 71)
4. **Aerobic capacity**
   6-minute walk test (page 150) *or*
   2-minute step-in-place test (page 153)
5. **Agility and dynamic balance**
   8-feet up-and-go test (page 221)

References

Miller, D. K. (2006). *Measurement by the physical educator: Why and how* (5th ed.). New York: McGraw-Hill.

Morrow, J. R., Jackson, A. W., Disch, J. G., & Mood, D. P. (2005). *Measurement and evaluation in human performance* (3rd ed.). Champaign, IL: Human Kinetics.

Rikli, R. E., & Jones, C. J. (1997). Assessing physical performance in independent older adults: Issues and guidelines. *Journal of Aging and Physical Activity, 5*(3), 244–261.

Rikli, R. E., & Jones, C. J. (1999). Development and validation of a functional fitness test for community-residing older adults. *Journal of Aging and Physical Activity, 7*(2), 129–161.

Rikli, R. E., & Jones, C. J. (1999). Functional fitness normative scores for community-residing older adults, ages 60–94. *Journal of Aging and Physical Activity, 7*(2), 162–181.

Rikli, R. E., & Jones, C. J. (2001). *Senior fitness test manual.* Champaign, IL: Human Kinetics.

■ NFL (AMERICAN FOOTBALL) TEST BATTERY

Objective: Measure the physical abilities of football athletes

Age Range: 18 to 35

Test Components:

1. **Muscular endurance**
   NFL-225 bench press test (page 50)
2. **Muscular power**
   Standing broad jump (page 110)
   Vertical jump (page 112)
3. **Speed and acceleration**
   40-yard dash test (page 224)
   3-cone drill (page 212)
   30-second chair stand test (page 71)
4. **Anaerobic capacity**
   60-yard shuttle test (page 178)

References

Inside the Combine. (2008, February 20). *Chicago Tribune,* 5–7.

Kuzmits, F. E., & Adams, A. J. (2008). The NFL Combine: Does it predict performance in the National Football League? *Journal of Strength and Conditioning Research, 22*(6), 1721–1727.

McGee, K. J., & Burkett, L. N. (2003). The National Football League Combine: A reliable predictor of draft status. *Journal of Strength and Conditioning Research, 17*(1), 6–11.

Sierer, S. P., Battaglini, C. L., Mihalik, J. P., Shields, E. W., & Tomasini, N. T. (2008). The National Football League Combine: Performance differences between drafted and nondrafted players entering the 2004 and 2005 drafts. *Journal of Strength and Conditioning Research, 22*(1), 6–12.

CHAPTER

2

Body Composition

Skinfold measurements are a practical method of estimating body composition in the field. Body composition is the amount of an individual's body mass that is composed of water, protein, minerals (fat-free mass), and fat, which is recorded as the relative body fat (%BF). Body composition is an indicator of overall health. There are other (laboratory) methods of estimating body composition (hydrostatic weighting, air displacement plethysmography, and DEXA scans) that are not discussed in this book. These methods require additional equipment and are typically not performed in the field. Skinfold measurements can be as accurate as the laboratory methods if the correct protocols and procedures are followed.

When utilizing skinfold measurements it is important the test administrator be sufficiently trained and practiced in the techniques of skinfold measurements. It is recommended that the test administrator perform at least 50 to 100 skinfold measurements under the direct supervision of an experienced examiner to become accustomed to the proper techniques. Skinfold measurements obtained from under-experienced examiners may result in higher measurement errors than those obtained by an experienced examiner.

Skinfold measurements are made with skinfold calipers and should be made on the test subject's *right* side. Differences exist between high-quality metal calipers and plastic calipers. It is generally recommended that high-quality metal calipers be utilized because they are more accurate while proving a more constant amount of tension. No matter which type of skinfold calipers are utilized, they should be calibrated and in proper working order. The test administrator should be comfortable and practiced with using the available calipers. The same skinfold calipers should be utilized on subsequent skinfold measurements made on the same test subject.

Before taking the skinfold measurements, the test administrator must first determine and physically mark (on each test subject) the proper location where the measurement will be taken from. This requires making marks on the test subject with a pen *before* skinfold measurements are obtained. Some skinfold measurement sites also require a small tape measure or ruler.

The test administrator also should determine which equation will be utilized. There are many separate equations to choose from. Each equation has been developed on and validated for a specific population based on age, gender, ethnicity, and activity level. Which equation is chosen determines the specific skinfold measurement sites the test administrator will measure. Utilizing an equation for a population for which it is not intended will result in calculation errors regardless of the test administrator's ability to properly use the skinfold techniques. Some common skinfold equations for athletes and physically active people are given at the end of this chapter (**Table 2-1**). The references listed are good sources for more specific information about skinfold measurements, as well as for where more skinfold measurement equations and formulas can be found.

■ CHEST/PECTORAL SKINFOLD SITE

Direction of Fold: Diagonal

Anatomical Reference: Axilla and nipple

Measurement Technique: The fold between the axilla and nipple is taken as high as possible on the anterior fold (**Figure 2-1**). The skinfold measurement is taken 1 centimeter below the test administrator's fingers.

References

American College of Sports Medicine. (2008). *ACSM's health-related physical fitness assessment manual* (2nd ed.). Atlanta: Lippincott Williams & Wilkins.

Heyward, V. H. (2006). *Advanced fitness assessment and exercise prescription* (5th ed.). Champaign, IL: Human Kinetics.

Heyward, V. H., & Wagner, D. R. (2004). *Applied body composition assessment* (2nd ed.). Champaign, IL: Human Kinetics.

Miller, D. K. (2006). *Measurement by the physical educator: Why and how* (5th ed.). New York: McGraw-Hill.

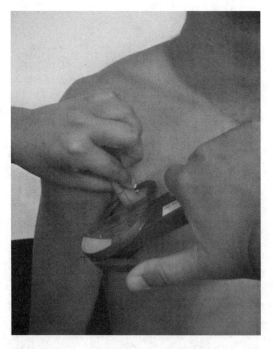

Figure 2-1   Chest/Pectoral Skinfold Site Measurement

■ SUBSCAPULAR SKINFOLD SITE

Direction of Fold: Diagonal

Anatomical Reference: Inferior angle of the scapula

Measurement Technique: The fold along the natural cleavage line of skin just below the inferior angle of the scapula is taken (**Figure 2-2**). The skinfold measurement is taken 1 centimeter below the test administrator's fingers.

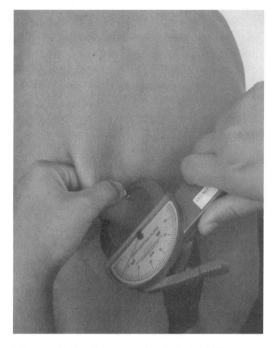

Figure 2-2   Subscapular Skinfold Site Measurement

References

American College of Sports Medicine. (2008). *ACSM's health-related physical fitness assessment manual* (2nd ed.). Atlanta: Lippincott Williams & Wilkins.

Carling, C., Reilly, T., & Williams, A. M. (2009). *Performance assessment for field sports.* New York: Routledge.

Heyward, V. H. (2006). *Advanced fitness assessment and exercise prescription* (5th ed.). Champaign, IL: Human Kinetics.

Heyward, V. H., & Wagner, D. R. (2004). *Applied body composition assessment* (2nd ed.). Champaign, IL: Human Kinetics.

Miller, D. K. (2006). *Measurement by the physical educator: Why and how* (5th ed.). New York: McGraw-Hill.

■ MIDAXILLARY SKINFOLD SITE

Direction of Fold: Horizontal

Anatomical Reference: Xiphisternal junction (point at which the costal cartilage of ribs 5 and 6 articulates with the sternum); this is slightly above the inferior tip of the xiphoid process

Measurement Technique: The fold is taken on the midaxillary line at the level of the xiphisternal junction (**Figure 2-3**).

References

American College of Sports Medicine. (2008). *ACSM's health-related physical fitness assessment manual* (2nd ed.). Atlanta: Lippincott Williams & Wilkins.

Heyward, V. H. (2006). *Advanced fitness assessment and exercise prescription* (5th ed.). Champaign, IL: Human Kinetics.

Heyward, V. H., & Wagner, D. R. (2004). *Applied body composition assessment* (2nd ed.). Champaign, IL: Human Kinetics.

Miller, D. K. (2006). *Measurement by the physical educator: Why and how* (5th ed.). New York: McGraw-Hill.

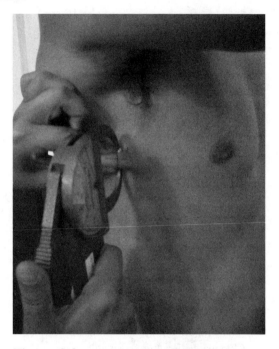

Figure 2-3   Midaxillary Skinfold Site Measurement

■ SUPRAILIAC SKINFOLD SITE

Direction of Fold: Oblique

Anatomical Reference: Iliac crest

Measurement Technique: The fold is taken posterior to the midaxilla line and superior to the iliac crest along the natural cleavage of skin (**Figure 2-4**). The skinfold measurement is taken 1 centimeter below the test administrator's fingers.

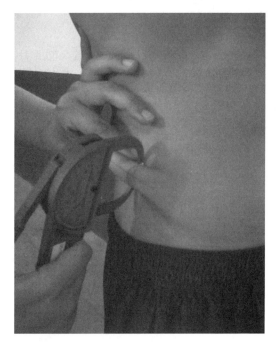

Figure 2-4   Suprailliac Skinfold Site Measurement

References

American College of Sports Medicine. (2008). *ACSM's health-related physical fitness assessment manual* (2nd ed.). Atlanta: Lippincott Williams & Wilkins.

Carling, C., Reilly, T., & Williams, A. M. (2009). *Performance assessment for field sports.* New York: Routledge.

Heyward, V. H. (2006). *Advanced fitness assessment and exercise prescription* (5th ed.). Champaign, IL: Human Kinetics.

Heyward, V. H., & Wagner, D. R. (2004). *Applied body composition assessment* (2nd ed.). Champaign, IL: Human Kinetics.

Miller, D. K. (2006). *Measurement by the physical educator: Why and how* (5th ed.). New York: McGraw-Hill.

ABDOMINAL SKINFOLD SITE

Direction of Fold: Horizontal

Anatomical Reference: Umbilicus

Measurement Technique: The fold is taken 3 centimeters lateral and 1 centimeter below the center of the umbilicus (**Figure 2-5**).

References

American College of Sports Medicine. (2008). *ACSM's health-related physical fitness assessment manual* (2nd ed.). Atlanta: Lippincott Williams & Wilkins.

Heyward, V. H. (2006). *Advanced fitness assessment and exercise prescription* (5th ed.). Champaign, IL: Human Kinetics.

Heyward, V. H., & Wagner, D. R. (2004). *Applied body composition assessment* (2nd ed.). Champaign, IL: Human Kinetics.

Miller, D. K. (2006). *Measurement by the physical educator: Why and how* (5th ed.). New York: McGraw-Hill.

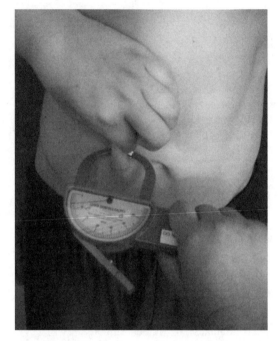

Figure 2-5 Abdominal Skinfold Site Measurement

TRICEPS SKINFOLD SITE

Direction of Fold: Vertical

Anatomical Reference: Acromion process (of scapula) and olecranon process of the ulna

Measurement Technique:

1. A tape measure is used to determine the distance between the lateral projection of the acromion process and the inferior margin of the olecranon process, as measured on the lateral aspect of the arm with the elbow flexed at 90° (**Figure 2-6**).

2. The midpoint is marked on the lateral side of the arm.

3. The fold is taken 1 centimeter above the mark. The skinfold measurement is taken at the marked point (**Figure 2-7**).

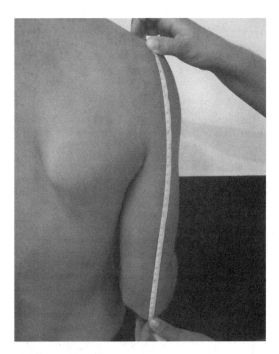

Figure 2-6 Measuring Placement of Triceps Skinfold Site

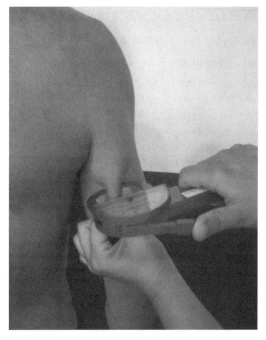

Figure 2-7 Triceps Skinfold Site Measurement

References

American College of Sports Medicine. (2008). *ACSM's health-related physical fitness assessment manual* (2nd ed.). Atlanta: Lippincott Williams & Wilkins.

Carling, C., Reilly, T., & Williams, A. M. (2009). *Performance assessment for field sports.* New York: Routledge.

Heyward, V. H. (2006). *Advanced fitness assessment and exercise prescription* (5th ed.). Champaign, IL: Human Kinetics.

Heyward, V. H., & Wagner, D. R. (2004). *Applied body composition assessment* (2nd ed.). Champaign, IL: Human Kinetics.

Miller, D. K. (2006). *Measurement by the physical educator: Why and how* (5th ed.). New York: McGraw-Hill.

■ BICEPS SKINFOLD SITE

Direction of Fold: Vertical

Anatomical Reference: Biceps brachii

Measurement Technique: The fold is taken over the biceps brachii at the level marked for the triceps on a line with the anterior border of the acrominion process and the antecubital fossa (**Figure 2-8**). The skinfold measurement is taken 1 centimeter below the test administrator's fingers.

References

American College of Sports Medicine. (2008). *ACSM's health-related physical fitness assessment manual* (2nd ed.). Atlanta: Lippincott Williams & Wilkins.

Carling, C., Reilly, T., & Williams, A. M. (2009). *Performance assessment for field sports.* New York: Routledge.

Heyward, V. H. (2006). *Advanced fitness assessment and exercise prescription* (5th ed.). Champaign, IL: Human Kinetics.

Heyward, V. H., & Wagner, D. R. (2004). *Applied body composition assessment* (2nd ed.). Champaign, IL: Human Kinetics.

Miller, D. K. (2006). *Measurement by the physical educator: Why and how* (5th ed.). New York: McGraw-Hill.

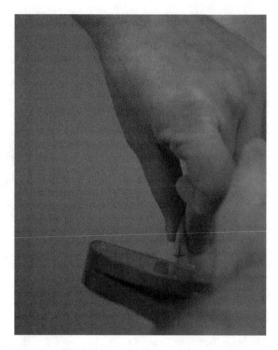

Figure 2-8   Biceps Skinfold Site Measurement

■ THIGH SKINFOLD SITE

Direction of Fold: Vertical

Anatomical Reference: Inguinal crease and patella

Measurement Technique: The test performer stands and places the right leg forward with the knee slightly bent. The fold on the anterior aspect of the thigh is taken midway between the inguinal crease and the proximal border of the patella. The test performer's body weight should shift to the opposite foot before the calipers are applied. The skinfold measurement is taken 1 centimeter below the test administrator's fingers (**Figure 2-9**).

References

American College of Sports Medicine. (2008). *ACSM's health-related physical fitness assessment manual* (2nd ed.). Atlanta: Lippincott Williams & Wilkins.

Carling, C., Reilly, T., & Williams, A. M. (2009). *Performance assessment for field sports.* New York: Routledge.

Heyward, V. H. (2006). *Advanced fitness assessment and exercise prescription* (5th ed.). Champaign, IL: Human Kinetics.

Heyward, V. H., & Wagner, D. R. (2004). *Applied body composition assessment* (2nd ed.). Champaign, IL: Human Kinetics.

Miller, D. K. (2006). *Measurement by the physical educator: Why and how* (5th ed.). New York: McGraw-Hill.

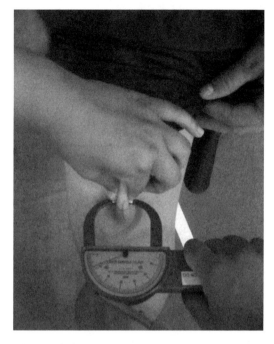

Figure 2-9   Thigh Skinfold Site Measurement

■ CALF SKINFOLD SITE

Direction of Fold: Vertical; on the medial calf

Anatomical Reference: Point of maximum calf circumference

Measurement Technique: The test performer sits on a chair or bench. The fold is taken at the level of maximum calf circumference on the medial aspect of the calf with the knee and hip flexed at 90° (**Figure 2-10**).

References

American College of Sports Medicine. (2008). *ACSM's health-related physical fitness assessment manual* (2nd ed.). Atlanta: Lippincott Williams & Wilkins.

Heyward, V. H. (2006). *Advanced fitness assessment and exercise prescription* (5th ed.). Champaign, IL: Human Kinetics.

Heyward, V. H., & Wagner, D. R. (2004). *Applied body composition assessment* (2nd ed.). Champaign, IL: Human Kinetics.

Miller, D. K. (2006). *Measurement by the physical educator: Why and how* (5th ed.). New York: McGraw-Hill.

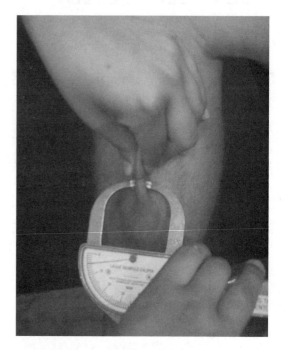

Figure 2-10   Calf Skinfold Site Measurement

■ BODY MASS INDEX (BMI)

Objective: Generally classify individuals as obese, overweight, or underweight and determine if an individual is at risk for obesity-related diseases; body mass index does not directly measure percentage of body fat

Age Range: All

Equipment Needed:

1. Calibrated scale
2. Tape measure

Additional Personnel Needed: None

Setup: The test performer removes his or her shoes and stands erect, preferably with the back against a wall.

Administration and Directions:

1. The test administrator measures the test performer's height with a tape measure or another accurate method. The test

performer should not be wearing shoes when his or her height is measured.

2. The test administrator weighs the test performer without his or her shoes while wearing a minimum of clothing to receive an accurate reading.

3. To calculate BMI, the test performer's height is converted to meters and weight converted to kilograms. Taking these measurements in meters and kilograms initially will avoid possible conversion errors.

Scoring:

1. Height is converted to meters.

$$\text{meters} = (\text{inches} \times 0.39) \div 100$$

2. Weight is converted to kilograms.

$$\text{kilograms} = \text{pounds} \div 2.2$$

3. The following calculation is performed and recorded as the final score.

$$\text{BMI} = \text{weight in kilograms} \div (\text{height in meters})^2$$

4. Alternatively, a nonogram can be utilized to calculate the BMI (**Figure 2-11**). To utilize the nonogram, a ruler is placed to connect the test performer's weight and height on the graph. The point where the ruler intersects the BMI column (middle column) is the BMI.

Checklist: The test performer must

1. Remove his or her shoes before the height and weight are measured
2. Stand erect when the height is measured
3. Wear a minimum of clothing when the weight is measured

References

American College of Sports Medicine. (2003). *ACSM's fitness book* (3rd ed.). Champaign, IL: Human Kinetics.

American College of Sports Medicine. (2008). *ACSM's health-related physical fitness assessment manual* (2nd ed.). Atlanta: Lippincott Williams & Wilkins.

Bray, G. A. (1978). Definition, measurement, and classification of the syndromes of obesity. *International Journal of Obesity, 2,* 99–112.

Carling, C., Reilly, T., & Williams, A. M. (2009). *Performance assessment for field sports.* New York: Routledge.

Heinrich, K. M., Jitnarin, N., Suminski, R. R., et al. (2008). Obesity classification in military personnel: A comparison of body fat, waist circumference, and body mass index measurements. *Military Medicine, 173,* 67–73.

Heyward, V. H., & Wagner, D. R. (2004). *Applied body composition assessment* (2nd ed.). Champaign, IL: Human Kinetics.

Kahn, H. S. (1991). A major error in nomograms for estimating body mass index. *American Journal of Clinical Nutrition, 54,* 435–437.

Miller, D. K. (2006). *Measurement by the physical educator: Why and how* (5th ed.). New York: McGraw-Hill.

Thomas, A. E., McKay, D. A., & Cutlip, M. B. (1976). A nomograph method for assessing body weight. *American Journal of Clinical Nutrition, 29,* 302–304.

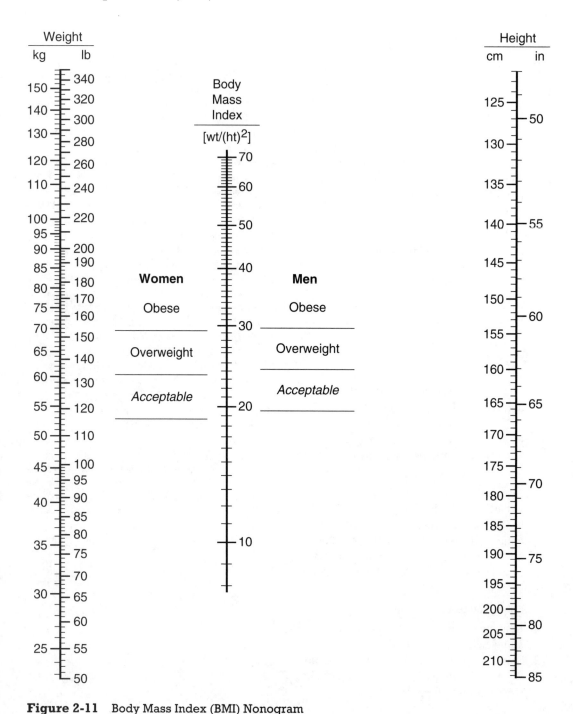

Figure 2-11 **Body Mass Index (BMI) Nonogram**
Source: Reprinted by permission from Macmillan Publishers Ltd. *International Journal of Obesity.* Bray, G. A.
Definition, measurement, and classification of the syndromes of obesity, vol. 2, pp. 99–112. Copyright 1978.

■ WAIST-TO-HIP RATIO (WHR)

Objective: Indirectly measure the difference between upper- and lower-body fat and weight distribution

Age Range: Child to adult

Equipment Needed:

1. Flexible tape measure

Additional Personnel Needed: None

Setup:

1. The test performer should be wearing a minimum of clothing.
2. The test performer stands erect.

Administration and Directions:

1. The test administrator measures the test performer's waist at the narrowest point between the inferior ribs and the iliac crest. This is generally approximately 2.5 centimeters (1 inch) above the navel (**Figure 2-12**).
2. The test administrator should measure the test performer's waist directly on the skin.
3. The test administrator measures the test performer's hips at the widest point of the buttocks. This is above the gluteal fold (**Figure 2-13**).
4. The test administrator should measure the test performer's hips with the tape measure directly on the skin or over only one layer of tight-fitting clothes.

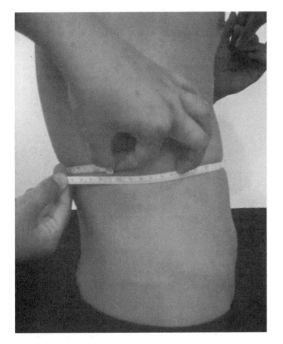

Figure 2-12 Waist Measurement Site

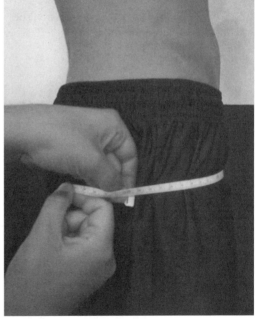

Figure 2-13 Hip Measurement Site

Scoring:

1. The test administrator records the waist and hip circumferences in centimeters.
2. The WHR is calculated by dividing the waist circumference (WC) by the hip circumference (HC) and recorded as the final score.

$$WHR = WC \div HC$$

3. Alternatively, a nonogram can be used to calculate the WHR (**Figure 2-14**). Place a ruler on the graph to connect the test performer's waist and hip circumferences. The point at which the ruler intersects the WHR column (middle column) indicates the WHR.

Checklist: The test performer must

1. Not pull in the stomach when the waist circumference is measured
2. Wear just one layer of clothing when the hip circumference is measured

References

American College of Sports Medicine. (2003). *ACSM's fitness book* (3rd ed.). Champaign, IL: Human Kinetics.

American College of Sports Medicine. (2008). *ACSM's health-related physical fitness assessment manual* (2nd ed.). Atlanta: Lippincott Williams & Wilkins.

Bray, G. A., & Gray, D. S. (1988). Obesity: Part 1—Pathogenesis. *Western Journal of Medicine, 149,* 429–441.

Carling, C., Reilly, T., & Williams, A. M. (2009). *Performance assessment for field sports.* New York: Routledge.

Heyward, V. H., & Wagner, D. R. (2004). *Applied body composition assessment* (2nd ed.). Champaign, IL: Human Kinetics.

Miller, D. K. (2006). *Measurement by the physical educator: Why and how* (5th ed.). New York: McGraw-Hill.

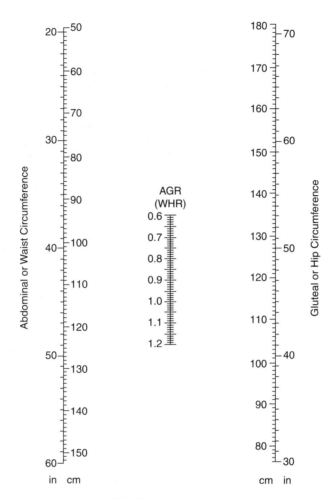

Figure 2-14   Waist-to-Hip Ratio (WHR) Nonogram

Source: Reproduced from *Western Journal of Medicine*, Bray, G. A., & Gray, D. S. Obesity: Part 1—
Pathogenesis. 1988, vol. 149, pp. 429–441. Reprinted with permission from the BMJ Publishing Group.

Table 2-1 Body Fat Equations for Selected Populations

FITNESSGRAM®/ACTIVITYGRAM® (Grades K–12)

Boys: %BF = 0.735($\sum 2$ skinfold) + 1.0

Girls: %BF = 0.610($\sum 2$ skinfold) + 5.1

$\sum 2$ skinfold = sum of skinfold from triceps and calf skinfold sites

Sources: Meredith, M. D., & Welk, C. J. (2007). *FITNESSGRAM®/ACTIVITYGRAM® test administration manual* (4th ed.). Champaign, IL: Human Kinetics.
Heyward, V. H., & Stolarczyk, L. M. (1996). *Applied body composition assessment.* Champaign, IL: Human Kinetics.

YMCA Physical Fitness Test

Men: %BF = 0.29288($\sum 4$ skinfold) − 0.0005($\sum 4$ skinfold)^2 + 0.15845(age) − 5.76377

Women: %BF = 0.29669($\sum 4$ skinfold) − 0.00043($\sum 4$ skinfold)^2 + 0.2963(age) + 1.4072

$\sum 4$ skinfold = total body fat from abdomen, ilium, triceps, and thigh skinfold sites

Source: Golding, L. A. (2000). *YMCA fitness testing and assessment manual* (4th ed.). Champaign, IL: Human Kinetics.

Athletes

Boys (14–19 years old): body density = 1.10647 − 0.00162(subscaplar skinfold) − 0.00144(abdominal skinfold) − 0.00077(triceps skinfold) + 0.00071(midaxillary skinfold)

Boys (13–16 years old): %BF = [(5.07 ÷ body density) − 4.5] × 100

Boys (17–19 years old): %BF = [(4.99 ÷ body density) − 4.55] × 100

Men (18–29 years old): body density = 1.112 − 0.00043499($\sum 7$ skinfold) + 0.00000055 ($\sum 7$ skinfold)^2 − 0.00028826(age)

$\sum 7$ skinfold = sum of skinfold from chest, midaxillary, subscapular, triceps, anterior suprailiac, abdomen, and thigh

Men: %BF = [(4.95 ÷ body density) − 4.5] × 100

Women (18–29 years old): body density = 1.096095 − 0.0006952($\sum 4$ skinfold) + 0.0000011 ($\sum 4$ skinfold)^2 − 0.0000714(age)

$\sum 4$ skinfold = sum of skinfold from triceps, anterior suprailiac, abdomen, and thigh

Women: %BF = [(5.01 ÷ body density) − 4.57] × 100

Source: Heyward, V. H., & Stolarczyk, L. M. (1996). *Applied body composition assessment.* Champaign, IL: Human Kinetics.

CHAPTER

3

Flexibility Testing

Flexibility is the range of motion possible about a joint. There are two separate types of flexibility that can be measured: absolute flexibility and relative flexibility. Absolute flexibility is the measurement of a joint in relation to a performance goal (i.e., total inches flexed forward). Relative flexibility is the measurement of a joint in relation to another measurement or body part (i.e., total inches flexed forward compared with body height).

The test administrator must ensure that all test performers who will perform flexibility testing properly warm up and stretch before the test is conducted. The test performer should slowly move into the stretched position and hold the final stretched position for several seconds while the test administrator scores the trial. The final stretched position should not result in the test performer experiencing any pain or excessive discomfort. The test administrator should ensure that the joint(s) being tested are properly isolated and the test performer is not cheating during the test or trial. If the test performer has an acute or chronic injury to the area to be flexibility tested, the test may need to be adjusted or not performed for safety reasons. Flexibility tests should be conducted at the beginning of any test battery.

■ SIT-AND-REACH TEST

Also Known as: Trunk Flexion Test

Objective: Measure static flexibility of the lower back, hip, and hamstring musculature

Age Range: 5 to adult

Equipment Needed:

1. Sit-and-reach box (commercially available) *or*
2. A box with a 12-inch (30.5-centimeter) cube and a measuring stick secured to the top
3. Wall

Additional Personnel Needed: None

Setup:

1. The 9-inch (23-centimeter) line on the slide ruler should be placed at the vertical section of the box.
2. The box is placed against a wall to prevent slippage.
3. The test performer removes his or her shoes.
4. The test performer sits with the knees straight and feet firmly placed against the vertical section of the box shoulder width apart (**Figure 3-1**).

Administration and Directions:

1. With the hands on top of each other and the palms down, the test performer leans forward (pushing the slide ruler on the box) slowly two to four times and holds the final attempt for 2 seconds (**Figure 3-2**).
2. Three trials are performed.

Scoring:

1. The most distant mark attained by the test performer is recorded as the final score.
2. A mark does not count if the test performer
   a. Bends the knees
   b. Reaches with the hands unevenly
   c. Does not hold the final position for 2 seconds

Checklist: The test performer must

1. Warm up properly before beginning the test
2. Remove his or her shoes
3. Keep the knees in an extended position (the test administrator may need to place the test performer's hands or a board on top of the knees to keep them straight)

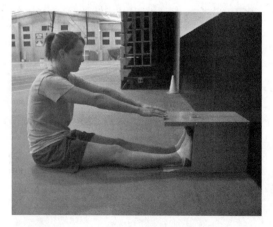

Figure 3-1 Sit-and-Reach Test Setup

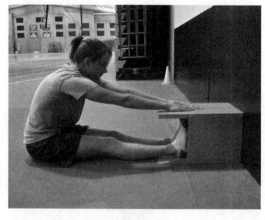

Figure 3-2 Sit-and-Reach Test Administration

4. Hold the final position for a minimum of 2 seconds
5. Not reach unevenly with the hands

References

American Alliance for Health, Physical Education, Recreation, and Dance (AAHPERD). (1980). *Lifetime health related physical fitness.* Reston, VA: AAHPERD.

American College of Sports Medicine. (2003). *ACSM's fitness book* (3rd ed.). Champaign, IL: Human Kinetics.

American College of Sports Medicine. (2008). *ACSM's health-related physical fitness assessment manual* (2nd ed.). Atlanta: Lippincott Williams & Wilkins.

Baltaci, G., Un, N., Tunay, V., Besler, A., & Gerçeker, S. (2003). Comparison of three different sit and reach tests for measurement of hamstring flexibility in female university students. *British Journal of Sports Medicine, 37*(1), 59–61.

Brodie, D. A. (1996). *A reference manual for human performance measurement in the field of physical education and sports sciences.* Lewiston, NY: Edwin Mellen.

Hartman, J. G., & Looney, M. (2003). Norm-referenced and criterion-referenced reliability and validity of the back-saver sit-and-reach. *Measurement in Physical Education and Exercise Science, 7*(2), 71–87.

Hoeger, W. W. K., Hopkins, D. R., Button, S., & Palmer, T. R. (1990). Comparing the sit and reach with the modified sit and reach in measuring flexibility in adolescents. *Pediatric Exercise Science, 2*, 156–162.

Hopkins, D. R., & Hoeger, W. W. K. (1992). A comparison of the sit-and-reach test and the modified sit-and-reach test in the measurement of flexibility for males. *Journal of Applied Sport Science Research, 6*(1), 7–10.

Hui, S. S. C., & Yuen, P. Y. (2000). Validity of the modified back-saver sit-and-reach test: A comparison with other protocols. *Medicine and Science in Sports and Exercise, 32*(9), 1655–1659.

Johnson, B. L., & Nelson, J. K. (1986). *Practical measurements for evaluation in physical education* (4th ed.). New York: MacMillan.

Liemoh, W., Sharpe, G. L., & Wasserman, J. F. (1994). Criterion related validity of the sit-and-reach test. *Journal of Strength and Conditioning Research, 8*(2), 91–94.

Martin, S. B., Jackson, A. W., & Morrow, J. R. (1998). The rationale for the sit and reach test revisited. *Measurement in Physical Education and Exercise Science, 2*(2), 85–92.

Prentice, W. E. (1997). *Fitness for college and life* (5th ed.). St. Louis: Mosby.

Roetert, E. P., Brown, S. W., Piorkowski, P. A., & Woods, R. B. (1996). Fitness comparisons among three different levels of elite tennis players. *Journal of Strength and Conditioning Research, 10*(3), 139–143.

Simoneau, G. G. (1998). The impact of various anthropometric and flexibility measurements on the sit-and-reach test. *Journal of Strength and Conditioning Research, 12*(4), 232–237.

Thorndyke, M. A. (1995). Evaluating flexibility with the sit and reach test. *Strength and Conditioning, 17*(6), 12–15.

Trehearn, T. L., & Buresh, R. J. (2009). Sit-and-reach flexibility and running economy of men and women collegiate distance runners. *Journal of Strength and Conditioning Research, 23*(1), 158–162.

Wells, K. F., & Dillon, E. K. (1952). The sit and reach—A test of back and leg flexibility. *Research Quarterly, 23*, 115–118.

■ MODIFIED SIT-AND-REACH TEST

Objective: Measure static flexibility of the lower back, hip, and hamstring musculature while controlling for arm and leg length

Age Range: 5 to adult

Equipment Needed:

1. Sit-and-reach box (commercially available) *or*
2. Box with a 12-inch (30.5-centimeter) cube and a measuring stick secured to the top
3. Wall

Additional Personnel Needed: Test assistant

Setup:

1. The test performer removes his or her shoes and sits against the wall with the head, back, and hips against the wall at a 90° angle. The knees should be straight and shoulder width apart.
2. The box is placed firmly against the test performer's feet, and the slide ruler on the box is pushed away from the test performer's body. A test assistant may need to secure the box so that it does not lose contact with the test performer's feet (**Figure 3-3**).

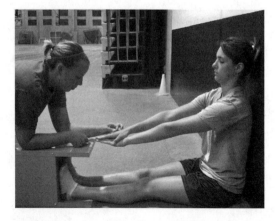

Figure 3-3   Modified Sit-and-Reach Test Setup

Administration and Directions:

1. With the hands on top of each other and the palms down, the test performer leans forward slowly *while keeping the head, back, and hips* against the wall at a 90° angle with the knees straight. When the test performer has reached as far as possible while keeping the body in the correct position, the test administrator moves the slide ruler until it touches the test performer's fingers. This distance is the finger-to-box distance (FBD) and will be used as the 0 measurement for scoring. If the test performer can not reach the ruler while keeping the head, back, and hips against the wall at a 90° angle, the test administrator will need to measure the distance with a tape measure and utilize this figure as the 0 measurement.
2. After the 0 measurement has been established, the test performer is allowed to perform a standard sit-and-reach test (see page 24) by leaning forward slowly with the hands on top of each other, palms down, and knees straight two to four times and holds the final attempt for 2 seconds (**Figure 3-4**). This is the reach distance (RD).
3. Three trials are performed.

Scoring:

1. The greatest RD attained by the test performer is documented.
2. The test administrator takes the RD and subtracts the FBD measurement.

$$RD - FBD$$

3. The resultant distance is recorded as the final score.

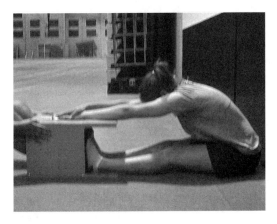

Figure 3-4 Modified Sit-and-Reach Test Administration

Checklist: The test performer must

1. Warm up properly before beginning the test
2. Remove his or her shoes
3. Keep the knees in an extended position (the test administrator may need to place the test performer's hands or a board on top of the knees to keep them straight)
4. Hold the final position for a minimum of 2 seconds
5. Not reach unevenly with the hands

References

Chung, P. K., & Yuen, C. K. (1999). Criterion-related validity of sit-and-reach tests in university men in Hong Kong. *Perceptual and Motor Skills, 88,* 204–316.

Heyward, V. H. (2006). *Advanced fitness assessment and exercise prescription* (5th ed.). Champaign, IL: Human Kinetics.

Hoeger, W. W. K., & Hopkins, D. R. (1992). A comparison of the sit and reach and the modified sit and reach in the measurement of flexibility in women. *Research Quarterly, 63*(2), 191–195.

Hoeger, W. W. K., Hopkins, D. R., Button, S., & Palmer, T. R. (1990). Comparing the sit and reach with the modified sit and reach in measuring flexibility in adolescents. *Pediatric Exercise Science, 2,* 156–162.

Hopkins, D. R., & Hoeger, W. W. K. (1992). A comparison of the sit-and-reach test and the modified sit-and-reach test in the measurement of flexibility for males. *Journal of Applied Sport Science Research, 6*(1), 7–10.

Hui, S. S. C., & Yuen, P. Y. (2000). Validity of the modified back-saver sit-and-reach test: A comparison with other protocols. *Medicine and Science in Sports and Exercise, 32*(9), 1655–1659.

Johnson, B. L., & Nelson, J. K. (1986). *Practical measurements for evaluation in physical education* (4th ed.). New York: MacMillan.

Lemmink, K. A., Kemper, H. C. G., Mathieu, H. G., Rispens, P., & Stevens, M. (2003). The validity of the sit-and-reach test and the modified sit-and-reach test in middle-aged to older men and women. *Research Quarterly for Exercise and Sport, 74*(3), 331–336.

Minkler, S., & Patterson, P. (1994). The validity of the modified sit-and-reach test in college-age students. *Research Quarterly for Exercise Science, 65*(2), 189–192.

■ YMCA SIT-AND-REACH TEST

Objective: Measure static flexibility of the lower back and hamstring musculature

Age Range: 5 to adult

Equipment Needed:

1. Measuring stick
2. Tape
3. Floor

Additional Personnel Needed: None

Setup:

1. The measuring stick is secured to the floor with tape perpendicular to the stick at the 15-inch (38-centimeter) mark. If a measuring stick is not available, a long strip of tape marked off with the distance can be utilized.
2. The test performer removes his or her shoes and sits with the measuring stick between the legs with the knees extended.
3. The test performer's heels should touch the edge of the taped perpendicular line with the heels 10 to 12 inches (25 to 30 centimeters) apart (**Figure 3-5**).

Administration and Directions:

1. With the hands on top of each other and the palms down, the test performer leans forward slowly two to four times and holds the final attempt for 2 seconds (**Figure 3-6**).
2. Three trials are performed.

Scoring:

1. The greatest distance attained by the test performer is recorded as the final score.
2. A mark does not count if the test performer
   a. Bends the knees
   b. Reaches with the hands unevenly
   c. Does not hold the final position for 2 seconds

Checklist: The test performer must

1. Warm up properly before beginning the test
2. Remove his or her shoes before beginning the test

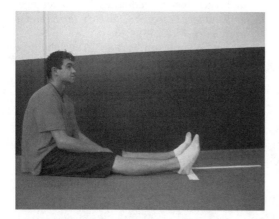

Figure 3-5   YMCA Sit-and-Reach Test Setup

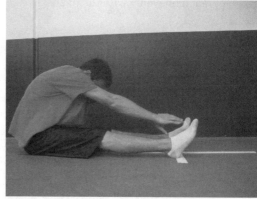

Figure 3-6   YMCA Sit-and-Reach Test Administration

3. Keep the knees in an extended position (the test administrator may need to place the test performer's hands or a board on top of the knees to keep them straight)
4. Hold the final position for a minimum of 2 seconds
5. Not reach unevenly with the hands

References

American College of Sports Medicine. (2008). *ACSM's health-related physical fitness assessment manual* (2nd ed.). Atlanta: Lippincott Williams & Wilkins.

Chung, P. K., & Yuen, C. K. (1999). Criterion-related validity of sit-and-reach tests in university men in Hong Kong. *Perceptual and Motor Skills, 88*, 204–316.

Golding, L. A. (2000). *YMCA fitness testing and assessment manual* (4th ed.). Champaign, IL: Human Kinetics.

■ SIT-AND-REACH WALL TEST

Objective: Provide a quick estimation of lower back and hamstring flexibility; multiple individuals may be tested simultaneously

Age Range: Middle school to college age

Equipment Needed:

1. Wall
2. Flat floor

Additional Personnel Needed: None

Setup:

1. The test performer removes his or her shoes and places the feet flat against the wall shoulder width apart (**Figure 3-7**).

Administration and Directions:

1. With the knees straight, the test performer reaches forward toward the wall with the objective of touching the wall with the fingertips, knuckles, or palms (**Figure 3-8**).
2. The test performer holds the final position for 3 seconds.
3. Three trials can be performed.

Scoring:

1. The following scoring criteria are based on which part of the test performer's hand is held against the wall for 3 seconds and is recorded as the final score.

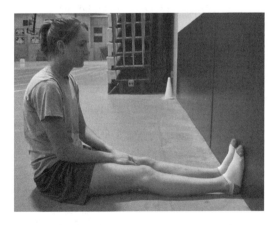

Figure 3-7 Sit-and-Reach Wall Test Setup

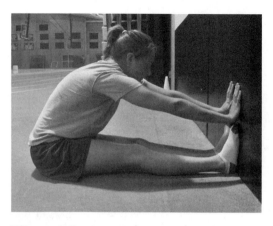

Figure 3-8 Sit-and-Reach Wall Test Administration

Palms: Excellent
Knuckles: Good
Fingertips: Average
Cannot touch the wall: Poor

Checklist: The test performer must

1. Keep the knees straight
2. Remove his or her shoes
3. Hold the final position for 3 seconds

Reference

Miller, D. K. (2006). *Measurement by the physical educator: Why and how* (5th ed.). New York: McGraw-Hill.

■ V-SIT-AND-REACH TEST

Objective: Measure static flexibility of the lower back and hamstring musculature

Age Range: 9 to 17

Equipment Needed:

1. Tape measure or measuring stick
2. Floor tape
3. Flat floor
4. Marking pen

Additional Personnel Needed: Test assistant

Setup:

1. A 2-foot (60-centimeter) baseline is created on the floor with tape.
2. At the midpoint of the baseline, place a 4-foot (1.2-meter) perpendicular taped line (measuring line) intersecting the baseline and extending 2 feet (0.6 meters) on each side of the baseline.
3. The measuring line is marked off in inches or centimeters.
4. The test performer removes his or her shoes and sits on the floor with the measuring line between the legs and the soles of the feet immediately behind the baseline 8 to 12 inches (20 to 30 centimeters) apart (**Figure 3-9**).

Administration and Directions:

1. The test performer keeps the knees straight and places the palms down on the measuring line.
2. The test performer keeps the knees straight and slowly reaches forward as far as possible (**Figure 3-10**).
3. The test performer has three practice (warm-up) trials.

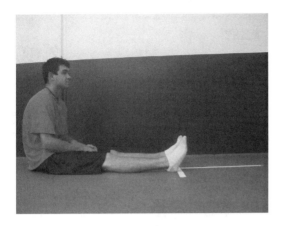

Figure 3-9 V-Sit-and-Reach Test Setup

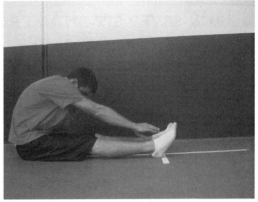

Figure 3-10 V-Sit-and-Reach Test Administration

4. On the fourth trial, the final position is held for 3 seconds while the test administrator records the distance.
5. A test assistant may be needed to keep the test performer's knees straight and the feet behind the baseline during the test.

Scoring:

1. The distance reached is recorded as the final score.
2. A mark does not count if the test performer
   a. Bends the knees
   b. Reaches with the hands unevenly
   c. Does not hold the final position for 3 seconds
   d. Slides the body or feet past the baseline

Checklist: The test performer must

1. Remove his or her shoes
2. Keep the knees straight
3. Hold the final position for 3 seconds

References

Baumgartner, T. A., Jackson, A. S., Mahar, M. T., & Rowe, D. A. (2007). *Measurement for evaluation in physical education and exercise science* (8th ed.). New York: McGraw-Hill.

Heyward, V. H. (2006). *Advanced fitness assessment and exercise prescription* (5th ed.). Champaign, IL: Human Kinetics.

Hui, S. S. C., & Yuen, P. Y. (2000). Validity of the modified back-saver sit-and-reach test: A comparison with other protocols. *Medicine and Science in Sports and Exercise, 32*(9), 1655–1659.

Miller, D. K. (2006). *Measurement by the physical educator: Why and how* (5th ed.). New York: McGraw-Hill.

Safrit, M. J. (1995). *Complete guide to youth fitness testing.* Champaign, IL: Human Kinetics.

■ BACK-SAVER SIT-AND-REACH TEST

Objective: Measure static flexibility of the lower back and hamstring musculature without causing excessive stress on the lower back

Age Range: 5 to 60+

Equipment Needed:

1. Sit-and-reach box (commercially available) *or*
2. Box with a 12-inch (30.5-centimeter) cube and a yard/meter stick secured to the top
3. Wall

Additional Personnel Needed: None

Setup:

1. The 9-inch (23-centimeter) line on the slide ruler should be placed at the vertical section of the box.
2. The box is placed against a wall to prevent slippage.
3. The test performer removes his or her shoes.

4. The test performer sits with the test leg straight and the foot firmly against the vertical section of the box in line with the shoulder (**Figure 3-11**).
5. The non-test knee is bent with the sole of the foot flat on the floor 2 to 3 inches (5 to 7.5 centimeters) away from the test knee.

Administration and Directions:

1. With the hands on top of each other and the palm down, the test performer leans forward slowly two to four times (pushing the slide ruler on the box), holding the final attempt for 2 seconds (**Figure 3-12**).
2. The test performer then switches legs, assumes the same relative position, and performs the test on the opposite side.
3. It is acceptable for the non-test foot to move slightly laterally when the body is flexed forward.
4. Up to three trials can be performed on each leg.

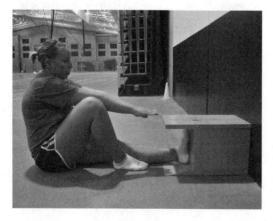

Figure 3-11 Back-Saver Sit-and-Reach Test Setup

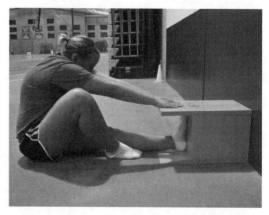

Figure 3-12 Back-Saver Sit-and-Reach Test Administration

Scoring:

1. The distance reached is recorded, to a maximum of 12 inches (30.5 centimeters), as the final score for each leg.
2. A mark does not count if the test performer
   a. Bends the knees
   b. Reaches with the hands unevenly
   c. Does not hold the stretched position for 2 seconds

Checklist: The test performer must

1. Remove his or her shoes
2. Keep the test knee straight and the non-test knee bent, with the foot flat on the floor
3. Hold the final position for 2 seconds

References

Baltaci, G., Un, N., Tunay, V., Besler, A., & Gerçeker, S. (2003). Comparison of three different sit and reach tests for measurement of hamstring flexibility in female university students. *British Journal of Sports Medicine, 37*(1), 59–61.

Baumgartner, T. A., Jackson, A. S., Mahar, M. T., & Rowe, D. A. (2007). *Measurement for evaluation in physical education and exercise science* (8th ed.). New York: McGraw-Hill.

Hartman, J. G., & Looney, M. (2003). Norm-referenced and criterion-referenced reliability and validity of the back-saver sit-and-reach. *Measurement in Physical Education and Exercise Science, 7*(2), 71–87.

Heyward, V. H. (2006). *Advanced fitness assessment and exercise prescription* (5th ed.). Champaign, IL: Human Kinetics.

Hui, S. S. C., & Yuen, P. Y. (2000). Validity of the modified back-saver sit-and-reach test: A comparison with other protocols. *Medicine and Science in Sports and Exercise, 32*(9), 1655–1659.

López-Miñarro, P. A., Baranda Andújar, P.S., & Rodríguez-García, P. L. (2009). A comparison of the sit-and-reach test and the back-saver sit-and-reach test in university students. *Journal of Sports Science and Medicine, 8,* 116–122.

Martin, S. B., Jackson, A. W., & Morrow, J. R. (1998). The rationale for the sit and reach test revisited. *Measurement in Physical Education and Exercise Science, 2*(2), 85–92.

Meredith, M. D., & Welk, C. J. (2007). *FITNESS-GRAM®/ACTIVITYGRAM® test administration manual* (4th ed.). Champaign, IL: Human Kinetics.

Miller, D. K. (2006). *Measurement by the physical educator: Why and how* (5th ed.). New York: McGraw-Hill.

Patterson, P., Wiksten, D. L., Ray, L., Flanders, C., & Sanphy, D. (1996). The validity and reliability of the back-saver sit-and-reach test in middle school girls and boys. *Research Quarterly for Exercise and Sport, 67*(4), 448–451.

Safrit, M, J. (1995). *Complete guide to youth fitness testing.* Champaign, IL: Human Kinetics.

■ MODIFIED BACK-SAVER SIT-AND-REACH TEST

Objective: Measure static flexibility of the lower back and hamstring musculature with minimal equipment without causing excessive stress on the lower back

Age Range: 5 to 60+

Equipment Needed:

1. Measuring stick
2. 12-inch (30.5-centimeter) bench
3. Tape

Additional Personnel Needed: Test assistant

Setup:

1. The measuring stick is secured to the top of the bench with the tape.
2. The test performer removes his or her shoes and sits on the bench with one leg straight (the test leg) and the opposite

(non-test) leg bent at a 90° angle with the foot flat on the floor (**Figure 3-13**).

Administration and Directions:

1. The test performer places the palms down on, or next to, the measuring stick.
2. The test performer keeps the test knee straight and slowly reaches forward as far as possible (**Figure 3-14**).
3. The test performer has three practice (warm-up) trials, and on the fourth trial the final position is held for 3 seconds while the test administrator records the distance.
4. The test performer then switches legs and follows the same protocol on the opposite leg.

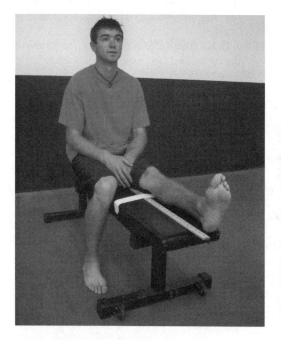

Figure 3-13   Modified Back-Saver Sit-and-Reach Test Setup

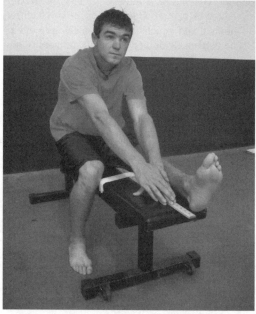

Figure 3-14   Modified Back-Saver Sit-and-Reach Test Administration

5. A test assistant may be needed to assist in securing the test performer on the bench or to ensure that the test performer keeps the test leg straight.
6. Up to three trials can be performed on each leg.

Scoring:

1. The distance reached is recorded as the final score for each leg.
2. A mark does not count if the test performer
   a. Bends the test knee
   b. Reaches with the hands unevenly
   c. Does not hold the final stretched position for 3 seconds
   d. Slides the body or feet past the baseline.

Checklist: The test performer must

1. Remove his or her shoes
2. Keep the test knee straight
3. Have the non-test leg bent at 90°, with the foot flat on the floor
4. Hold the final position for 3 seconds

References

Heyward, V. H. (2006). *Advanced fitness assessment and exercise prescription* (5th ed.). Champaign, IL: Human Kinetics.

Hui, S. S. C., & Yuen, P. Y. (2000). Validity of the modified back-saver sit-and-reach test: A comparison with other protocols. *Medicine and Science in Sports and Exercise, 32*(9), 1655–1659.

■ CHAIR SIT-AND-REACH TEST

Objective: Measure static flexibility of the hamstring musculature in an elderly subject

Age Range: 60 to 90+

Equipment Needed:

1. Tape measure or measuring stick
2. Straight back or folding chair
3. Wall

Additional Personnel Needed: None

Setup:

1. The chair is placed against a wall or otherwise secured.
2. The test performer sits on the front edge of the chair. The crease between the buttocks and thigh should be even with the edge of the chair.
3. The test performer determines a preferred leg. The preferred leg is the one that is believed will result in a better score. This is the leg that is extended and tested.
4. The knee of the non-preferred leg is bent and the foot placed flat on the floor.
5. The knee of the preferred leg is extended straight in front of the hip with the heel on the floor and the foot dorsiflexed to approximately 90°.
6. The test performer places the hands palms down and on top of each other with the middle fingers even (**Figure 3-15**).

Administration and Directions:

1. The test performer keeps the preferred leg straight (but not hyperextended) and slowly bends forward *at the hip*, sliding the hands down the preferred leg, attempting to touch their toes (**Figure 3-16**).

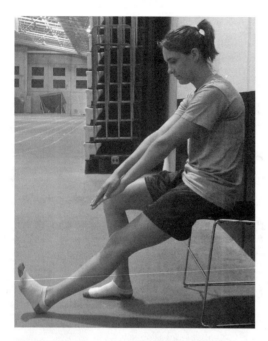

Figure 3-15 Chair Sit-and-Reach Test Setup

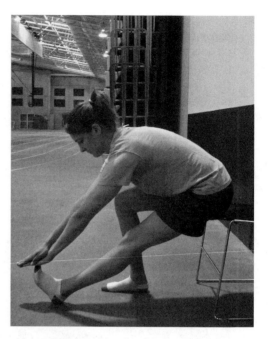

Figure 3-16 Chair Sit-and-Reach Test Administration

2. The test performer's spine should remain straight with the head in line with the spine (not tucked) as the hands move forward.
3. The farthest reach is held for 2 seconds while the test administrator measures the trial.
4. Two practice trials are given before the two test trials.

Scoring:

1. A test performer who can touch and hold the toe at the end of the shoe receives a score of 0.
2. For every inch the test performer is able to reach and hold past the toe, a positive score is received to the nearest half-inch. For example, a score of 3 is given if the test performer can reach 3 inches beyond the toe.

3. For every inch the test performer is short of reaching the toe, a negative score is received to the nearest half-inch. For example, a score of –3 is given if the test performer is 3 inches short of reaching the toe.
4. The farthest distance reached is recorded as the final score.

Checklist: The test performer must

1. Keep the dominant knee straight while flexing forward at the hip
2. Exhale while flexing forward
3. Keep the spine straight and the head in line with the spine while flexing forward
4. Avoid bouncing, rapid, forceful movements and stretching to the point of pain
5. Hold the final stretch position for a minimum of 2 seconds

References

Baltaci, G., Un, N., Tunay, V., Besler, A., & Gerçeker, S. (2003). Comparison of three different sit and reach tests for measurement of hamstring flexibility in female university students. *British Journal of Sports Medicine*, *37*(1), 59–61.

Baumgartner, T. A., Jackson, A. S., Mahar, M. T., & Rowe, D. A. (2007). *Measurement for evaluation in physical education and exercise science* (8th ed.). New York: McGraw-Hill.

Cavani, V., Mier, C. M., Musto, A. A., & Tummers, N. (2002). Effects of a 6-week resistance-training program on functional fitness of older adults. *Journal of Aging and Physical Activity, 10,* 443–452.

Jones, C. J., Rikli, R. E., Max, J., & Noffal, G. (1998). The reliability and validity of a chair sit-and-reach test as a measure of hamstring flexibility in older adults. *Research Quarterly for Exercise and Sport, 69*(4), 338–343.

Morrow, J. R., Jackson, A. W., Disch, J. G., & Mood, D. P. (2005). *Measurement and evaluation in human performance* (3rd ed.). Champaign, IL: Human Kinetics.

Rikli, R. E., & Jones, C. J. (1999). Development and validation of a functional fitness test for community-residing older adults. *Journal of Aging and Physical Activity, 7,* 129–161.

Rikli, R. E., & Jones, C. J. (1999). Functional fitness normative scores for community-residing older adults, ages 60–94. *Journal of Aging and Physical Activity, 7,* 162–182.

Rikli, R. E., & Jones, C. J. (2001). *Senior fitness test manual.* Champaign, IL: Human Kinetics.

■ TRUNK LIFT TEST

Also Known as: Trunk Extension Test

Objective: Measures absolute extension flexibility of the trunk

Age Range: 6 to college age

Equipment Needed:

1. Exercise mat
2. Tape measure or measuring stick

Additional Personnel Needed: Test assistant

Setup:

1. The test performer lies prone on the exercise mat and interlaces the fingers behind the head.
2. The test assistant secures the test performer's hips against the exercise mat (**Figure 3-17**).

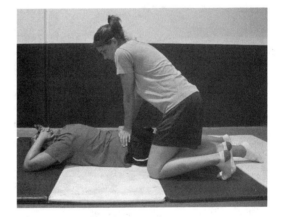

Figure 3-17 Trunk Extension Test Setup

Administration and Directions:

1. On the test administrator's "go" command, the test performer raises the chest and head in a controlled manner off the exercise mat as far as possible (**Figure 3-18**).
2. The head should be kept in line with the spine and should not hyperextend.
3. The final position is held until the test administrator can take the measurement.
4. The test performer should not be encouraged to lift higher than 12 inches (30.5 centimeters) off the exercise mat.
5. Three trials are performed.

Scoring:

1. The distance from the test performer's chin to the exercise mat is measured.
2. The farthest measurement is recorded as the final score.

Checklist: The test performer must

1. Have the hips securely held to the exercise mat by the test assistant

2. Keep the fingers interlaced behind the head
3. Keep the head in line and not hyperextend the head
4. Not experience back discomfort; if the performer does, the test should be stopped immediately

References

Anderson, B. (1981). Conditioning report: Flexibility testing. *National Strength Coaches Association Journal, 3*(2), 20–23.

Baumgartner, T. A., Jackson, A. S., Mahar, M. T., & Rowe, D. A. (2007). *Measurement for evaluation in physical education and exercise science* (8th ed.). New York: McGraw-Hill.

Hannibal, N. S., Plowman, S. A., Looney, M. A., & Brandenburg, J. (2006). Reliability and validity of low back strength/muscular field tests in adolescents. *Journal of Physical Activity and Health, 3*(Supplement 2), S78–S89.

Jackson, A. W., Morrow, J. R., Jensen, R. L., Jones, N. A., & Schultes, S. S. (1996). Reliability of the Prudential FITNESSGRAM™ trunk lift test in young adults. *Research Quarterly for Exercise and Sport, 67*(1), 115–117.

Meredith, M. D., & Welk, C. J. (2007). *FITNESSGRAM®/ACTIVITYGRAM® test administration manual* (4th ed.). Champaign, IL: Human Kinetics.

Miller, D. K. (2006). *Measurement by the physical educator: Why and how* (5th ed.). New York: McGraw-Hill.

Prentice, W. E. (1997). *Fitness for college and life* (5th ed.). St. Louis: Mosby.

Safrit, M. J. (1995). *Complete guide to youth fitness testing*. Champaign, IL: Human Kinetics.

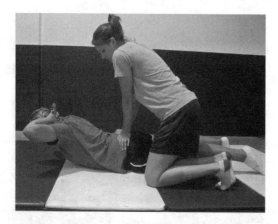

Figure 3-18 Trunk Extension Test Administration

■ TRUNK-AND-NECK EXTENSION TEST

Objective: Measure relative extension flexibility of the trunk

Age Range: 6 to college age

Equipment Needed:

1. Exercise mat
2. Tape measure or measuring stick
3. Chair

Additional Personnel Needed: Test assistant

Setup:

1. The test performer sits in the chair, keeping the chin level.
2. The test administrator measures the distance from the tip of the test performer's nose to the chair. This is the trunk-and-neck-length measurement and will be utilized during scoring (**Figure 3-19**).
3. The test performer then lies prone on the exercise mat with the hands on the lower back.
4. The test assistant secures the test performer's hips against the exercise mat (**Figure 3-20**).

Administration and Directions:

1. On the test administrator's "go" command, the test performer slowly raises the chest and head in a controlled manner off the exercise mat as far as possible (**Figure 3-21**).
2. The head may hyperextend during this test.
3. The final position is held until the test administrator can take the measurement; this is the trunk-lift measurement.
4. Three trials are performed.

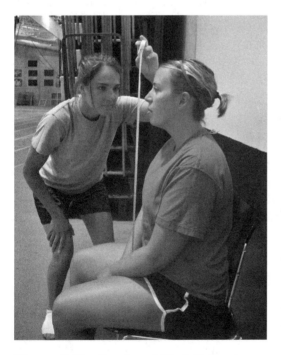

Figure 3-19 Trunk-and-Neck Extension Test Measurement

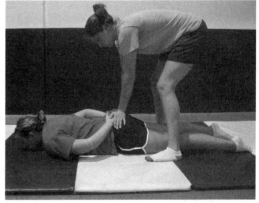

Figure 3-20 Trunk-and-Neck Extension Test Setup

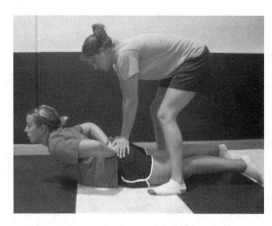

Figure 3-21 Trunk-and-Neck Extension Test Administration

Scoring:

1. The distance from the tip of the test performer's chin to the exercise mat is measured.
2. The final score is the trunk-and-neck length subtracted from the best trunk-lift measurement.

trunk lift – trunk-and-neck length

3. The closer the trunk lift is to the trunk-and-neck-length measurement, the better the score.

Checklist: The test performer must

1. Have the hips securely held to the exercise mat by the test assistant
2. Keep the hands on the lower back
3. Not experience back discomfort; if the performer does, the test should be stopped immediately

References

Johnson, B. L., & Nelson, J. K. (1986). *Practical measurements for evaluation in physical education* (4th ed.). New York: MacMillan.

Nakanishi, Y., & Nethery, V. (1998). Physiological and fitness comparison between young Japanese and American males. *Journal of Physiological Anthropology and Applied Human Science, 17*(5), 189–193.

Miller, D. K. (2006). *Measurement by the physical educator: Why and how* (5th ed.). New York: McGraw-Hill.

■ SHOULDER LIFT TEST

Objective: Measure absolute flexibility of the shoulder

Age Range: 6 to college age

Equipment Needed:

1. Exercise mat
2. Two measuring sticks *or*
3. One measuring stick and one tape measure

Additional Personnel Needed: None

Setup:

1. The test performer lies prone with the chin on the exercise mat and arms extended forward directly in front of the shoulder.

2. The test performer is given a measuring stick to be held by both hands parallel to the shoulders at shoulder width apart (**Figure 3-22**).

Administration and Directions:

1. On the test administrator's "go" command, the test performer raises both shoulders while keeping the elbows and wrists straight and the chin on the exercise mat (**Figure 3-23**).
2. The test performer maintains the lifted position until the test administrator can take the measurement using either another measuring stick or a tape measure.
3. Three trials are performed.

Scoring:

1. The distance from the middle of the measuring stick to the exercise mat is measured.

2. The greatest distance is recorded as the final score.

Checklist: The test performer must

1. Keep the chin on the exercise mat
2. Keep the elbows and wrists straight when the shoulders are lifted

References

Baumgartner, T. A., Jackson, A. S., Mahar, M. T., & Rowe, D. A. (2007). *Measurement for evaluation in physical education and exercise science* (8th ed.). New York: McGraw-Hill.

Miller, D. K. (2006). *Measurement by the physical educator: Why and how* (5th ed.). New York: McGraw-Hill.

Prentice, W. E. (1997). *Fitness for college and life* (5th ed.). St. Louis: Mosby.

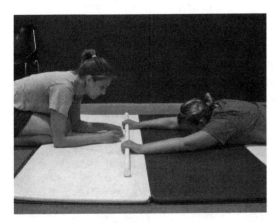

Figure 3-22   Shoulder Lift Test Setup

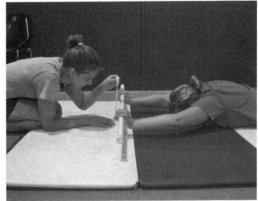

Figure 3-23   Shoulder Lift Test Administration

■ SHOULDER-AND-WRIST ELEVATION TEST

Objective: Measure relative shoulder and wrist flexibility

Age Range: 6 to college age

Equipment Needed:

1. Exercise mat
2. Two measuring sticks *or*
3. One measuring stick and one tape measure

Additional Personnel Needed: None

Setup:

1. With the test performer standing and the arms hanging at the side, the test administrator measures the test performer's arm length from the acromion

process to the tip of the middle finger (**Figure 3-24**). This represents the arm-length measurement and will be used during scoring.

2. The test performer lies prone with the chin on the exercise mat and the arms extended forward directly in front of the shoulders.
3. The test performer is given a measuring stick to be held by both hands parallel to the shoulders at shoulder width apart (**Figure 3-25**).

Administration and Directions:

1. On the test administrator's "go" command, the test performer raises both shoulders while keeping the elbows straight and the chin on the exercise mat.
2. The wrists may hyperextend during this test.
3. The test performer maintains the lifted position until the test administrator measures the trial (**Figure 3-26**).
4. Three trials are performed.

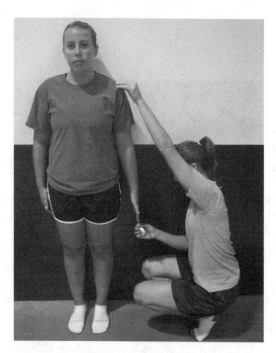

Figure 3-24 Shoulder-and-Wrist Elevation Test Measurement

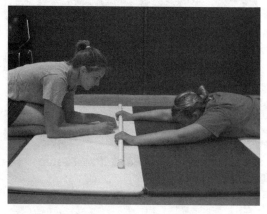

Figure 3-25 Shoulder-and-Wrist Elevation Test Setup

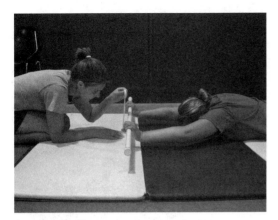

Figure 3-26 Shoulder-and-Wrist Elevation Test Administration

Scoring:

1. The distance from the top of the measuring stick to the exercise mat is measured.
2. The final score is the distance of the best trial subtracted from the arm-length measurement.

shoulder elevation – arm-length measurement

3. The closer the shoulder elevation is to the arm-length measurement, the better the score.

Checklist: The test performer must

1. Keep the chin on the exercise mat
2. Keep the elbows straight when the shoulders are lifted
3. Not experience back discomfort; if the performer does, the test must be stopped immediately

References

Johnson, B. L., & Nelson, J. K. (1986). *Practical measurements for evaluation in physical education* (4th ed.). New York: MacMillan.

Miller, D. K. (2006). *Measurement by the physical educator: Why and how* (5th ed.). New York: McGraw-Hill.

■ BACK SCRATCH TEST

Also Known as: Shoulder Stretch Test

Objective: Measure general static shoulder flexibility

Age Range: Child to 60+

Equipment Needed: Tape measure or ruler

Additional Personnel Needed: None

Setup:

1. The test performer stands and chooses a preferred hand (the hand that is believed will result in a better score).

2. The test performer's preferred hand is put over the same shoulder on the middle of the back with the palm down. The palm should touch the back.
3. The test performer's non-preferred hand is placed palm down in an opposite manner on the lower part of the back.
4. The test administrator examines the hands to determine if the test performer's middle fingers are approximately in alignment and makes adjustments if necessary (**Figure 3-27**).

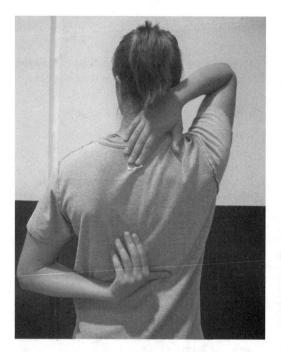

Figure 3-27 Back Scratch Test Setup

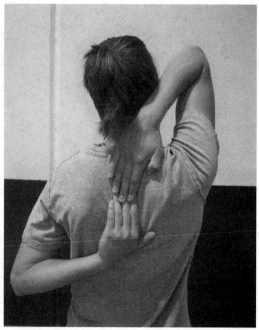

Figure 3-28 Back Scratch Test Administration

Administration and Directions:

1. On the test administrator's "go" command, the test performer brings the hands as close to each other as possible, overlapping the fingers if possible (**Figure 3-28**).
2. Two practice trials are performed before two test trials.

Scoring:

1. If the test performer can touch the tips of the middle fingers together, a score of 0 is given.
2. For every inch of overlap the test performer can create and hold with the middle fingers, a positive score is given to the nearest half-inch. For example, a score of 1 is given if the test performer can overlap the middle fingers by 1 inch.

3. For every inch that the test performer's middle fingers are short of touching, a negative score is given to the nearest half-inch. For example, a score of –1 is given if the test performer is short of overlapping the middle fingers by 1 inch.
4. The measurement is recorded as the final score.

Checklist: The test performer must

1. Keep the middle fingers in alignment before beginning to bring the hands together
2. Avoid forceful movements and stretching to the point of pain
3. Keep the hands in place until the test administrator can take the measurement

References

Annesi, J. J., Westcott, W. L., Faigenbaum, A. D., & Unruh, J. L. (2005). Effects of a 12-week physical activity protocol delivered by YMCA after-school counselors (Youth Fit for Life) on fitness and self-efficacy changes in 5–12-year-old boys and girls. *Research Quarterly for Exercise and Sport, 76*(4), 468–476.

Cavani, V., Mier, C. M., Musto, A. A., & Tummers, N. (2002). Effects of a 6-week resistance-training program on functional fitness of older adults. *Journal of Aging and Physical Activity, 10,* 443–452.

Meredith, M. D., & Welk, C. J. (2007). *FITNESSGRAM®/ACTIVITYGRAM® test administration manual* (4th ed.). Champaign, IL: Human Kinetics.

Miller, D. K. (2006). *Measurement by the physical educator: Why and how* (5th ed.). New York: McGraw-Hill.

Morrow, J. R., Jackson, A. W., Disch, J. G., & Mood, D. P. (2005). *Measurement and evaluation in human performance* (3rd ed.). Champaign, IL: Human Kinetics.

Rikli, R. E., & Jones, C. J. (1999). Development and validation of a functional fitness test for community-residing older adults. *Journal of Aging and Physical Activity, 7,* 129–161.

Rikli, R. E., & Jones, C. J. (1999). Functional fitness normative scores for community-residing older adults, ages 60–94. *Journal of Aging and Physical Activity, 7,* 162–182.

Rikli, R. E., & Jones, C. J. (2001). *Senior fitness test manual.* Champaign, IL: Human Kinetics.

Safrit, M. J. (1995). *Complete guide to youth fitness testing.* Champaign, IL: Human Kinetics.

CHAPTER 4

Local Muscular Endurance Testing

Local muscular endurance is the ability of a muscle or muscle group to resist fatigue by contracting continuously against a submaximal force. Local muscular endurance tests are related to strength testing and have many similar testing techniques, the primary difference being the amount of resistance utilized and the number of repetitions performed.

Local muscular endurance tests require the test performer to use proper techniques. Although the risk of acute or catastrophic injury from utilizing improper technique (from local muscular endurance testing) is less when compared with muscular strength testing, improper technique does result in the test performer fatiguing earlier than he or she otherwise may. The test administrator may require the test performer to warm up before a local muscular endurance test is conducted; excessive warming up, however, may result in a decreased score when the test is conducted. Local muscular endurance tests should be performed after agility, strength, and speed testing. If multiple local muscular endurance tests are performed on the same muscle groups during a single test battery, the tests should be separated by at least 5 minutes.

■ YMCA BENCH PRESS TEST

Objective: Evaluate endurance of the anterior upper arms, chest, and shoulder musculature

Age Range: High school to 60+

Equipment Needed:

1. Metronome
2. Weight rack (bench)
3. 35-pound (15.8-kilogram) barbell (for females)
4. 80-pound (36.2-kilogram) barbell (for males)

Additional Personnel Needed: Test assistant (spotter)

Setup:

1. The test administrator sets the metronome to 60 beats per minute (BPM).
2. The appropriate barbell is selected and placed on the weight rack.
   a. Females use a 35-pound (15.8-kilogram) barbell.
   b. Males use a 80-pound (36.2-kilogram) barbell.
3. The test performer assumes the proper bench press position by lying supine with both feet flat on the floor, grasping the bar with a closed, pronated grip slightly wider than shoulder width.
4. The test assistant assumes the proper bench press spotting position by standing behind the barbell at the test performer's head, grasping the bar with a closed, alternated grip inside the test performer's grip (**Figure 4-1**).
5. The test assistant and the test performer use proper communication to raise the barbell off the rack, and the weight is lowered to the test performer's chest. The barbell is resting on the test performer's chest with the elbows flexed (**Figure 4-2**). This is the starting position.

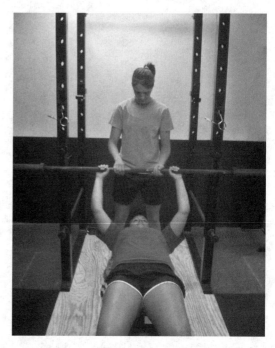

Figure 4-1   YMCA Bench Press Test Setup

6. The test performer may practice the protocol (described below) for a few repetitions to become accustomed to the pace and moving in rhythm with the metronome.

Administration and Directions:

1. On the test administrator's "go" command, the test performer presses the barbell up and down at the cadence of 30 repetitions per minute, utilizing proper bench press technique. Each time the metronome beeps, the test performer should move the barbell to the next position (up or down) (**Figure 4-3**).

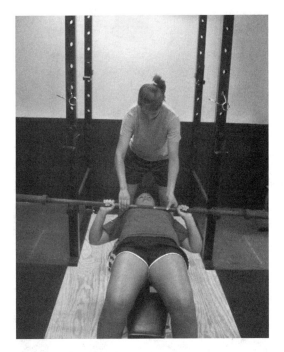

Figure 4-2   YMCA Bench Press Test
Starting Postion

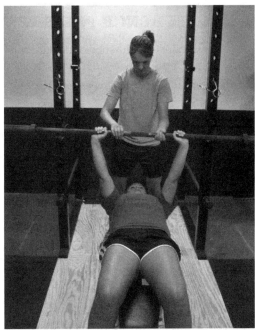

Figure 4-3   YMCA Bench Press Test
Administration

2. When the barbell is moved up, the test performer's elbows should be fully extended.
3. When the barbell is moved down, the test performer's elbows should be flexed, with the barbell returned to the starting position.
4. The test performer continues this process until the elbows cannot fully extend or the cadence can not be maintained.
5. One trial is performed.

Scoring:

1. Each time the test performer fully extends the elbows and returns the barbell to starting position at the designated cadence utilizing proper technique is counted as 1.
2. The final score is the total number of proper bench presses completed.

Checklist: The test performer must

1. Maintain proper bench press technique
2. Fully extend the elbows on each bench press attempt
3. Not move the bar faster or slower than the cadence
4. Utilize proper communication with the test assistant (spotter)

References

Baechle, T. R., & Earle, R. W. (2008). *Essentials of strength training and conditioning* (3rd ed.). Champaign, IL: Human Kinetics.

Golding, L. A. (2000). *YMCA fitness testing and assessment manual* (4th ed.). Champaign, IL: Human Kinetics.

Tritschler, K. (2000). *Barrow & McGee's practical measurement and assessment* (5th ed.). Philadelphia: Lippincott Williams & Wilkins.

■ NFL-225 BENCH PRESS TEST

Objective: Evaluate endurance of the anterior upper arms, chest, and shoulder musculature

Age Range: Adult (test for males only)

Equipment Needed:

1. Weight rack (bench)
2. 225 pounds (102 kilograms) of weight

Additional Personnel Needed: Test assistant (spotter)

Setup:

1. The test administrator puts 225 pounds (102 kilograms) on the weight rack.
2. The test performer assumes the proper bench press position by lying supine with both feet flat on the floor, grasping the bar with a closed, pronated grip slightly wider than shoulder width apart.
3. The test assistant assumes a proper bench press spotting position by standing behind the barbell at the test performer's head, grasping the bar with a closed, alternated grip inside the test performer's grip (**Figure 4-4**).
4. The test assistant and the test performer use proper communication to raise the barbell off the rack, and the weight is lowered to the test performer's chest. The barbell is resting on the test performer's chest with the elbows flexed (**Figure 4-5**). This is the starting position.

Administration and Directions:

1. On the test administrator's "go" command, the test performer presses the barbell up and down continuously, utilizing proper bench press technique at a pace of his choice (**Figure 4-6**).
2. When the barbell is moved up, the test performer's elbows should be fully extended.

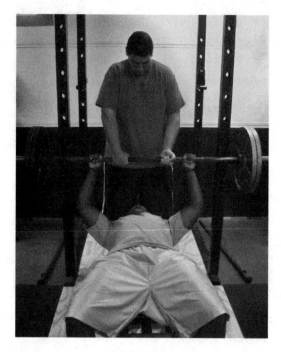

Figure 4-4 NFL-225 Bench Press Test Setup

3. When the barbell is moved down, the test performer's elbows should be flexed, with the barbell returned to the starting position.
4. The test performer is not required to keep a certain cadence during the test, but should be encouraged to keep a constant pace and not be allowed more than a two-second rest between repetition attempts when the weight is resting on the chest.
5. The test performer continues this process until exhaustion.
6. One trial is performed.

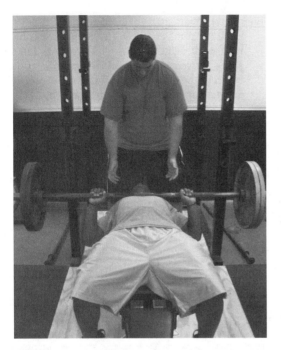

Figure 4-5 NFL-225 Bench Press Test Starting Positon

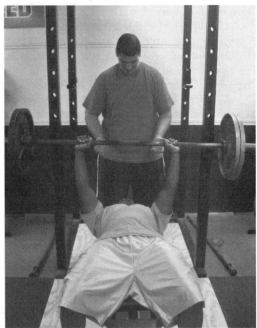

Figure 4-6 NFL-225 Bench Press Test Administration

Scoring:

1. Each time the test performer fully extends the elbows and returns the barbell to the starting position utilizing proper technique is counted as 1.
2. The final score is the total number of proper bench presses completed.

Checklist: The test performer must

1. Have good general upper-body strength, endurance, and bench press experience before attempting this test
2. Maintain a constant pace
3. Maintain proper bench press technique
4. Extend elbows fully for each bench press attempt
5. Utilize proper communication with the test assistant (spotter)
6. Not rest for more than 2 seconds between repetition attempts

References

Chapman, P. P., Whitehead, J. R., & Binkert, R. H. (1998). The 225-lb reps-to-fatigue test as a submaximal estimate of 1-RM bench press performance in college football players. *Journal of Strength and Conditioning Research, 12*(4), 258–261.

Inside the Combine. (2008, February 20). *Chicago Tribune,* 5–7.

Kuzmits, F. E., & Adams, A. J. (2008). The NFL Combine: Does it predict performance in the National Football League? *Journal of Strength and Conditioning Research, 22*(6), 1721–1727.

Mayhew, J. L., Jacques, J. A., Ware, J. S., Chapman, P. P., et al. (2004). Anthropometric dimensions do not enhance one repetition maximum prediction from the NFL-225 test in college football layers. *Journal of Strength and Conditioning Research.* 18(3), 572–578: 2004.

Mayhew, J. L., Ware, J. S., Bemben, M. G., Wilt, B., et al. (1999). The NFL-225 test as a measure of bench press strength in college football players. *Journal of Strength and Conditioning Research, 13*(2), 130–134.

Mayhew, J. L., Ware, J. S., Cannon, K., Corbett, S., et al. (2002). Validation of the NFL-225 test for predicting 1-RM bench press performance in college football players. *Journal of Sports Medicine and Physical Fitness, 42*(3), 304–308.

McGee, K. J., & Burkett, L. N. (2003). The National Football League Combine: A reliable predictor of draft status. *Journal of Strength and Conditioning Research, 17*(1), 6–11.

Sierer, S. P., Battaglini, C. L., Mihalik, J. P., Shields, E. W., & Tomasini, N. T. (2008). The National Football League Combine: Performance differences between drafted and nondrafted players entering the 2004 and 2005 drafts. *Journal of Strength and Conditioning Research, 22*(1), 6–12.

■ PULL-UPS FOR ENDURANCE TEST

Objective: Evaluate the endurance of the anterior arm and shoulder musculature

Age Range: 9 to college age

Equipment Needed:

1. Metal or wooden bar approximately 1.5 inches (3.8 centimeters) in diameter that is located (or can be adjusted) to a height that will not allow the test performer's feet to touch the ground.

Additional Personnel Needed: Test assistant

Setup:

1. The test performer jumps, or is aided by the test assistant, and grasps the bar with the palms forward (overhand grip) (**Figure 4-7**).
2. The test performer's feet should not touch the ground.
3. If the bar can not be adjusted to avoid having the feet touch the ground, the test performer should bend the knees and cross the feet during this test (**Figure 4-8**).

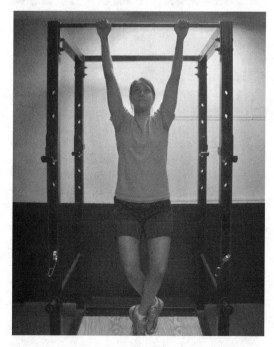

Figure 4-7 Pull-Ups for Endurance Test Setup

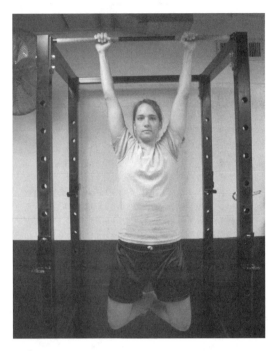

Figure 4-8 Pull-Ups for Endurance Test Alternative Setup

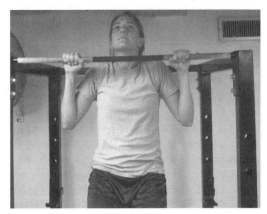

Figure 4-9 Pull-Ups for Endurance Test Administration

Administration and Directions:

1. On the test administrator's "go" command, the test performer pulls his or her body vertically until the chin is above the bar by flexing the elbows at a pace of his or her choice (**Figure 4-9**).
2. The test performer returns to the starting position.
3. The test performer completes as many pull-ups as possible without rest until exhaustion.
4. The test performer is not required to maintain a certain cadence during the test, but he or she should be encouraged to keep a constant pace and not rest excessively between pull-up attempts.
5. The test performer continues this process until exhaustion.
6. One trial is performed (unless it is obvious that the test performer can obtain a higher score, or loses his or her grip).

Scoring:

1. Each properly completed pull-up is counted as 1.
2. The total number of properly completed pull-ups is recorded as the final score.

Checklist: The test performer must

1. Not flex the hips
2. Extend the elbows fully between attempts
3. Not swing or kick the legs or lower body during the test

References

American Association for Health, Physical Education, Recreation, and Dance. (1976). *AAHPER youth fitness test manual.* Washington, DC: AAHPERD.

Coaches roundtable: Testing for football. (1983). *National Strength and Conditioning Association Journal,* 5(5), 12–19.

Brodie, D. A. (1996). *A reference manual for human performance measurement in the field of physical education and sports sciences.* Lewiston, NY: Edwin Mellen Press.

Heyward, V. H. (2006). *Advanced fitness assessment and exercise prescription* (5th ed.). Champaign, IL: Human Kinetics.

Johnson, B. L., & Nelson, J. K. (1986). *Practical measurements for evaluation in physical education* (4th ed.). New York: MacMillan.

LaChance, P. F., & Hortobagy, T. (1994). Influence of cadence on muscular performance during push-up and pull-up exercise. *Journal of Strength and Conditioning Research, 8*(2), 76–29.

McSwegin, P., Pemberton, C., Petray, C., & Going, S. (1989). *Physical best: The AAHPERD guide to physical fitness education and assessment.* Reston, VA: AAHPERD.

Meredith, M. D., & Welk, C. J. *FITNESSGRAM®/ ACTIVITYGRAM® test administration manual* (4th ed.). Champaign, IL: Human Kinetics.

Miller, D. K. (2006). *Measurement by the physical educator: Why and how* (5th ed.). New York: McGraw-Hill.

Rutherford, W. J., & Corbin, C. B. (1994). Validation of criterion-referenced standards for test of arm and shoulder girdle strength and endurance. *Research Quarterly for Exercise and Sport, 65*(2): 110–119.

Safrit, M. J. (1995). *Complete guide to youth fitness testing.* Champaign, IL: Human Kinetics.

Semenick, D., Connors, J., Carter, M., Harman, E., et al. (1992). Test and measurement: Rationale, protocols, testing/reporting forms and instructions for wrestling. *National Strength and Conditioning Association Journal, 14*(3), 54–59.

■ MODIFIED PULL-UPS FOR ENDURANCE TEST

Objective: Measure anterior arm and shoulder girdle endurance

Age Range: 10 to college age; this test is designed for females, but may be used for individuals who are unable to perform the pull-ups for endurance test

Equipment Needed: Adjustable horizontal bar

Additional Personnel Needed: None

Setup:

1. With the test performer standing next to the horizontal bar, the test administrator adjusts the horizontal bar, aligning it with the base of the test performer's sternum.

2. The test performer grasps the horizontal bar with the palms forward (overhand grip).

3. The test performer slides the feet under the horizontal bar until the arms are straight and the angle between the arms and trunk is 90° (**Figure 4-10**).

Administration and Directions:

1. On the test administrator's "go" command, the test performer flexes the elbows until the chin is raised over the horizontal bar, while keeping the body straight and rigid at a comfortable pace (**Figure 4-11**).

2. The test performer returns to the starting position.

3. The test performer continues this process until exhaustion.

4. The test performer is not required to maintain a certain cadence during the

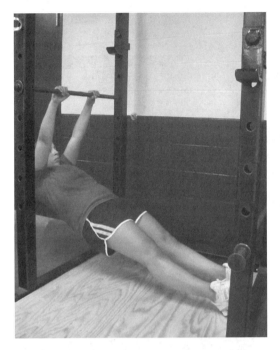

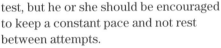

Figure 4-10   Modified Pull-Ups for Endurance Test Setup

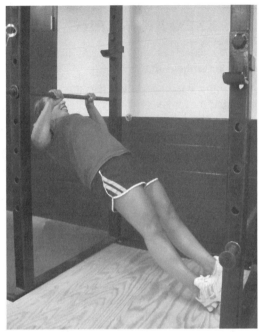

Figure 4-11   Modified Pull-Ups for Endurance Test Administration

test, but he or she should be encouraged to keep a constant pace and not rest between attempts.

5. One trial is performed (unless it is obvious that the test performer can obtain a higher score, or loses his or her grip).

Scoring:

1. Each properly completed modified pull-up is counted as 1.
2. The total number of properly completed modified pull-ups is recorded as the final score.

Checklist: The test performer must

1. Keep the body rigid
2. Extend the elbows fully between attempts
3. Not swing the body to generate momentum during the test

References

American College of Sports Medicine (2003). *ACSM's fitness book* (3rd ed.). Champaign, IL: Human Kinetics.

McSwegin, P., Pemberton, C., Petray, C., & Going, S. (1989). *Physical best: The AAHPERD guide to physical fitness education and assessment.* Reston, VA: AAHPERD.

Meredith, M. D., & Welk, C. J. *FITNESSGRAM®/ ACTIVITYGRAM® test administration manual* (4th ed.). Champaign, IL: Human Kinetics.

Miller, D. K. (2006). *Measurement by the physical educator: Why and how* (5th ed.). New York: McGraw-Hill.

Prentice, W. E. (1997). *Fitness for college and life* (5th ed.). St. Louis: Mosby.

Safrit, M. J. (1995). *Complete guide to youth fitness testing.* Champaign, IL: Human Kinetics.

■ FLEXED ARM-HANG TEST

Objective: Measure static anterior arm and shoulder girdle endurance

Age Range: 6 to college age; this test is designed for females but may be used for individuals who are unable to perform the pull-ups for endurance test

Equipment Needed:

1. Stopwatch
2. Horizontal bar 1.5 inches (3.8 centimeters) in diameter

Additional Personnel Needed: Two test assistants

Setup:

1. The test performer grasps the bar with the palms forward (overhand grip).
2. The test assistants help the test performer lift him- or herself off the floor high enough that the chin is above the horizontal bar and the elbows are flexed. The test assistants hold the test performer in this position until the test administrator gives the "go" command (**Figure 4-12**).
3. The test performer should not be able to touch the ground while in the flexed-arm position.
4. The test performer signals to the test administrator when ready.

Administration and Directions:

1. On the test administrator's "go" command, the test assistants release their support of the test performer.
2. The test performer keeps the chin above the horizontal bar as long as possible by utilizing only the arms (**Figure 4-13**).
3. One trial is performed (unless it is obvious that the test performer can

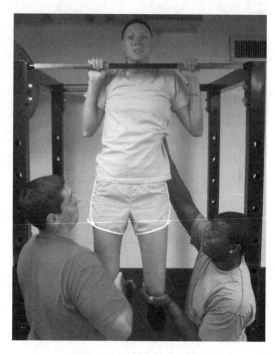

Figure 4-12 Flexed Arm-Hang Test Setup

obtain a higher score or loses his or her grip).

Scoring:

1. The test administrator begins timing the trial when the test assistants release the test performer, and stops timing the trial when the test performer's chin touches the bar, tilts backward, or drops below the horizontal bar.
2. The time is recorded as the final score.

Checklist: The test performer must

1. Not use the legs or feet for support during the test

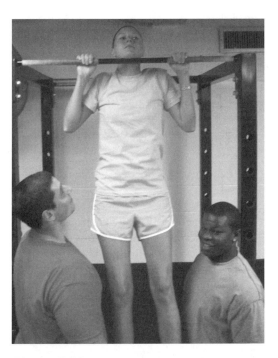

Figure 4-13 Flexed Arm-Hang Test Administration

2. Maintain the grip on the horizontal bar to avoid injury when completing the test
3. Signal the test assistants to release their support when he or she is ready

References

American Association for Health, Physical Education, Recreation, and Dance (AAHPERD). (1976). *AAHPER youth fitness test manual.* Washington, DC: AAHPERD.

Brodie, D. A. (1996). *A reference manual for human performance measurement in the field of physical education and sports sciences.* Lewiston, NY: Edwin Mellen Press.

Johnson, B. L., & Nelson, J. K. (1986). *Practical measurements for evaluation in physical education* (4th ed.). New York: MacMillan.

Meredith, M. D., & Welk, C. J. *FITNESSGRAM®/ACTIVITYGRAM® test administration manual* (4th ed.). Champaign, IL: Human Kinetics.

Miller, D. K. (2006). *Measurement by the physical educator: Why and how* (5th ed.). New York: McGraw-Hill.

Prentice, W. E. (1997). *Fitness for college and life* (5th ed.). St. Louis: Mosby.

Rutherford, W. J., & Corbin, C. B. (1994). Validation of criterion-referenced standards for test of arm and shoulder girdle strength and endurance. *Research Quarterly for Exercise and Sport, 65*(2), 110–119.

Safrit, M. J. (1995). *Complete guide to youth fitness testing.* Champaign, IL: Human Kinetics.

Tritschler, K. (2000). *Barrow & McGee's practical measurement and assessment* (5th ed.). Philadelphia: Lippincott Williams & Wilkins.

■ DIPS FOR ENDURANCE TEST

Objective: Measure posterior arm and shoulder girdle endurance

Age Range: 10 to college age

Equipment Needed: Parallel bars (adjustable)

Additional Personnel Needed: None

Setup:

1. The parallel bars are adjusted so that the test performer will not be in contact with the floor when lowering the body into the bent-arm position.

2. If the parallel bars cannot be adjusted, the test performer should bend the knees and cross the feet during this test.

3. The test performer grasps the bar and assumes a straight-arm position with elbows extended (**Figure 4-14**).

Administration and Directions:

1. On the test administrator's "go" command, the test performer lowers the body until the elbows are flexed at a 90° angle or less. This is the bent-arm position (**Figure 4-15**).

2. The test performer then returns to the straight-arm position (elbows extended).

3. The test performer continues this process until exhaustion.

4. The test performer is not required to maintain a certain cadence during the test, but he or she should be encouraged to keep a constant pace and not rest between attempts.

5. One trial is performed (unless it is obvious that the test performer can obtain a higher score, or loses his or her grip).

Scoring:

1. Each properly completed dip is counted as 1.

2. The total number of properly completed dips is recorded as the final score.

3. A dip does not count if the test performer
   a. Does not reach either the bent-arm or straight-arm position
   b. Touches the ground with the feet

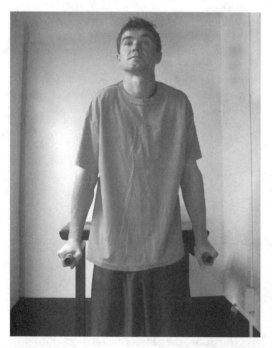

Figure 4-14   Dips for Endurance Test Setup

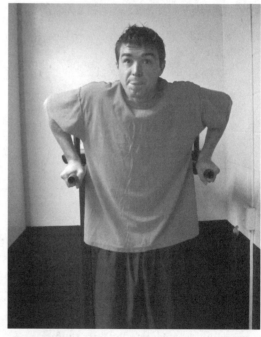

Figure 4-15   Dips for Endurance Test Administration

Checklist: The test performer must

1. Not touch the floor while performing this test
2. Lower the body until the elbows are flexed to at least a 90° angle
3. Not rest between dips
4. Not swing the body during the test

References

Coaches roundtable: Testing for football. (1983). *National Strength and Conditioning Association Journal, 5*(5), 12–19.

Johnson, B. L., & Nelson, J. K. (1986). *Practical measurements for evaluation in physical education* (4th ed.). New York: MacMillan.

Miller, D. K. (2006). *Measurement by the physical educator: Why and how* (5th ed.). New York: McGraw-Hill.

Semenick, D. (1981). Conditioning program: Testing and evaluation. *National Strength and Conditioning Association Journal, 3*(2): 8–9.

■ PUSH-UPS FOR ENDURANCE TEST

Objective: Evaluate the endurance of the upper arm, chest, and shoulder musculature

Age Range: 10 to college age

Equipment Needed:

1. Stopwatch
2. Flat, solid surface

Additional Personnel Needed: None

Setup:

1. The test performer assumes the proper push-up position with the face toward the floor, body straight, hands flat on the floor beneath the shoulders, elbows straight, toes on the ground. This is the starting (straight-arm) position (**Figure 4-16**).

Administration and Directions:

1. On the test administrator's "go" command, the test performer flexes the elbows until the chest touches the ground (**Figure 4-17**).

2. A thin piece of padding (or a sponge) may be placed on the floor underneath the test performer's chest to assist the performer in determining when the chest is on the ground.

3. The test performer then returns to the starting position.

4. The test performer completes as many push-ups as possible without rest for 1 minute.

5. The test performer is not required to maintain a certain cadence during the test, but he or she should be encouraged to keep a constant pace and not rest between attempts.

6. One trial is performed.

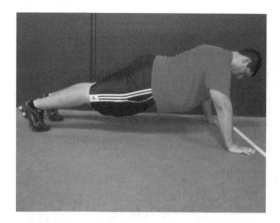

Figure 4-16   Push-Ups for Endurance Test Setup

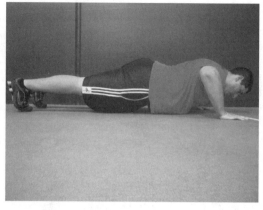

Figure 4-17   Push-Ups for Endurance Test Administration

Scoring:

1. Each properly completed push-up is counted as 1.
2. The total number of properly completed push-ups completed in 1 minute is recorded as the final score.

Checklist: The test performer must

1. Maintain the straight-body position (not pike or sag the spine)
2. Extend the elbows fully on each attempt
3. Lower the chest completely to the floor between repetitions
4. Not rest between push-ups

References

American College of Sports Medicine. (2003). *ACSM's fitness book* (3rd ed.). Champaign, IL: Human Kinetics.

American College of Sports Medicine. (2006). *ACSM's guidelines for exercise testing and prescription* (7th ed.). Philadelphia: Lippincott Williams & Wilkins.

Baechle, T. R., & Earle, R. W. (2008). *Essentials of strength training and conditioning* (3rd ed.). Champaign, IL: Human Kinetics.

Baumgartner, T. A., Oh, S., Chung, H., & Hales, D. (2002). Objectivity, reliability, and validity for a revised push-up test protocol. *Measurement in Physical Education and Exercise Science, 6*(4), 225–242.

Getchell, B., Mikesky, A. E., & Mikesky, K. N. (1998). *Physical fitness: A way of life* (5th ed.). Boston: Allyn and Bacon.

Gouvali, M. K., & Boudolos, K. (2005). Dynamic and electromyographical analysis variants of push-up exercise. *Journal of Strength and Conditioning Research, 19*(1), 146–151.

Heyward, V. H. (2006). *Advanced fitness assessment and exercise prescription* (5th ed.). Champaign, IL: Human Kinetics.

Johnson, B. L., & Nelson, J. K. (1986). *Practical measurements for evaluation in physical education* (4th ed.). New York: MacMillan.

LaChance, P. F., & Hortobagy, T. (1994). Influence of cadence on muscular performance during push-up and pull-up exercise. *Journal of Strength and Conditioning Research, 8*(2), 76–29.

Mayhew, J. L., Ball, T. E., Arnold, M. D., & Bowen, J. C. (1991). Push-ups as a measure of upper body strength. *Journal of Applied Sport Science Research, 5*(1), 16–21.

Meredith, M. D., & Welk, C. J. *FITNESSGRAM®/ACTIVITYGRAM® test administration manual* (4th ed.). Champaign, IL: Human Kinetics.

Prentice, W. E. (1997). *Fitness for college and life* (5th ed.). St. Louis: Mosby.

Roetert, E. P., Brown, S. W., Piorkowski, P. A., & Woods, R. B. (1996). Fitness comparisons among three different levels of elite tennis players. *Journal of Strength and Conditioning Research, 10*(3), 139–143.

Roetert, E. P., Garrett, G. E., Brown, S. W., & Camaione, D. N. (1992). Performance profiles of nationally ranked junior tennis players. *Journal of Applied Sport Science Research, 6*(4), 225–231.

Roetert, E. P., Piorkowski, P. A., Woods, R. B., & Brown, S. W. (1995). Establishing percentiles for junior tennis players based on physical fitness testing results. *Clinics in Sports Medicine, 14*(1), 1–21.

Rutherford, W. J., & Corbin, C. B. (1994). Validation of criterion-referenced standards for test of arm and shoulder girdle strength and endurance. *Research Quarterly for Exercise and Sport, 65*(2), 110–119.

Safrit, M. J. (1995). *Complete guide to youth fitness testing.* Champaign, IL: Human Kinetics.

Semenick, D., Connors, J., Carter, M., Harman, E., et al. (1992). Test and measurement: Rationale, protocols, testing/reporting forms and instructions for wrestling. *National Strength and Conditioning Association Journal, 14*(3), 54–59.

Tritschler, K. (2000). *Barrow & McGee's practical measurement and assessment* (5th ed.). Philadelphia: Lippincott Williams & Wilkins.

■ MODIFIED PUSH-UPS FOR ENDURANCE TEST

Also Known as: Bent Knee Push-Ups Test

Objective: Measure anterior arm and shoulder girdle endurance

Age Range: 10 to adult; this test is designed for females but may be used for individuals who are unable to perform the push-ups for endurance test

Equipment Needed:

1. Stopwatch
2. Flat, solid surface (floor)
3. Padding may be used for the test performer's knees

Additional Personnel Needed: None

Setup:

1. The test performer lies prone on the floor with the knees on the floor and the ankles at a 90° angle.

2. The test performer's body and trunk should be straight, with palms flat on the floor directly beneath the shoulders, and the elbows bent (**Figure 4-18**).

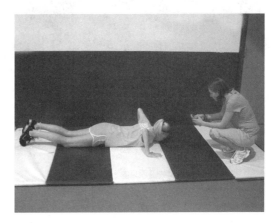

Figure 4-18   Modified Push-Ups for Endurance Test Setup

Administration and Directions:

1. On the test administrator's "go" command, the test performer extends the elbows, raising the body until the elbows are straight (**Figure 4-19**).
2. The test performer should keep the knees on the floor with the body and trunk straight.
3. The test performer then returns to the starting position.
4. The test performer completes as many modified push-ups as possible without rest for 1 minute.
5. The test performer is not required to maintain a certain cadence during the test, but he or should be encouraged to keep a constant pace and not rest between attempts.
6. One trial is performed.

Scoring:

1. Each properly completed modified push-up counts as 1.

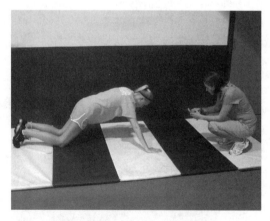

Figure 4-19 Modified Push-Ups for Endurance Test Administration

2. The total number of modified push-ups properly completed in 1 minute is recorded as the final score.

Checklist: The test performer must

1. Keep the body and trunk straight
2. Extend the elbows fully on each attempt
3. Lower the chest completely to the floor between repetitions
4. Not rest between modified push-ups

References

Baechle, T. R., & Earle, R. W. (2008). *Essentials of strength training and conditioning* (3rd ed.). Champaign, IL: Human Kinetics.

Johnson, B. L., & Nelson, J. K. (1986). *Practical measurements for evaluation in physical education* (4th ed.). New York: MacMillan.

Mayhew, J. L., Ball, T. E., Bowen, J. C., & Arnold, M. D. (1990). Pushups as a measure of upper body strength in females. *Journal of Osteopathic Sports Medicine, 4*(3), 11–14.

Miller, D. K. (2006). *Measurement by the physical educator: Why and how* (5th ed.). New York: McGraw-Hill.

Prentice, W. E. (1997). *Fitness for college and life* (5th ed.). St. Louis: Mosby.

Wood, H. M., & Baumgartner, T. A. (2004). Objectivity, reliability, and validity of the bent-knee push-up for college-aged women. *Measurement in Physical Education and Exercise Science, 8*(4), 203–212.

Safrit, M. J. (1995). *Complete guide to youth fitness testing.* Champaign, IL: Human Kinetics.

Suni, J. H., Oja, P., Miilunpalo, S. I., Pasanen, M. E., Vuori, I. M., & Bos, K. (1998). Health-related fitness test battery for adults: Associations with perceived health, mobility, and back function and symptoms. *Archives of Physical Medicine and Rehabilitation, 79,* 559–569.

■ ARM-CURL TEST

Objective: Measure anterior upper-arm muscle endurance

Age Range: 60 to 95+

Equipment Needed:

1. Stopwatch
2. Chair with a straight back and no arm rests
3. 5-pound (2.5-kilogram) dumbbell (for females)
4. 8-pound (3.6-kilogram) dumbbell (for males)

Additional Personnel Needed: Test assistant

Setup:

1. The test administrator asks the test performer which is his or her dominant hand (generally the hand used to write).
2. The test performer sits in the chair with the back straight and feet flat on the floor. The test performer's dominant side should be positioned toward the outside of the chair.
3. The test performer is given the proper dumbbell, and he or she holds it perpendicular to the floor with the elbow straight; the palm should face the body in the same manner in which the test performer shakes hands.
4. The test administrator assumes a position either behind or beside the test performer with his or her finger on the test performer's upper arm. The test administrator's fingers should be placed on the test performer's upper arm to prevent excessive upper-arm movement and ensure a full range of motion (**Figure 4-20**).
5. The test assistant should kneel on the same side where the test performer is holding the dumbbell.

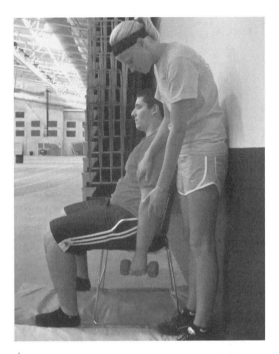

Figure 4-20   Arm-Curl Test Setup

6. The test performer is allowed to practice the proper arm-curl technique (described below) once or twice to become accustomed to the motion.

Administration and Directions:

1. On the test administrator's "go" command, the test performer flexes the elbow, raising the dumbbell toward the shoulder as far as possible (**Figure 4-21**).
2. As the dumbbell is curled, the test performer's palm should slowly rotate toward the ceiling (palm up) before returning to the starting position.
3. The test performer repeats this motion continuously for 30 seconds at a

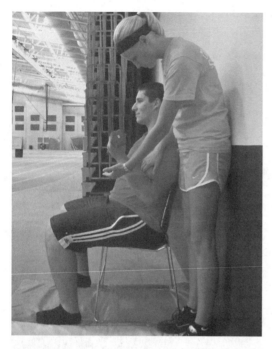

Figure 4-21 Arm-Curl Test Administration

comfortable, self-directed, and constant pace.

4. The test administrator or test assistant may be needed to remove the weight from the test performer during the test to prevent injury.

5. One trial is performed.

Scoring:

1. The final score is the total number of proper arm curls completed in 30 seconds.

2. If the test performer has curled the dumbbell more than halfway upward when the time elapses, it is considered a complete arm curl.

Checklist: The test performer must

1. Extend and flex the elbow fully during the curling motion and rotate the forearm properly during each arm curl
2. Not move the shoulder or swing the arm during the motion
3. Perform the test at a comfortable and constant pace

References

Cavani, V., Mier, C. M., Musto, A. A., & Tummers, N. (2002). Effects of a 6-week resistance-training program on functional fitness of older adults. *Journal of Aging and Physical Activity, 10*, 443–452.

Morrow, J. R., Jackson, A. W., Disch, J. G., & Mood, D. P. (2005). *Measurement and evaluation in human performance* (3rd ed.). Champaign, IL: Human Kinetics.

Rikli, R. E., & Jones, C. J. (1999). Development and validation of a functional fitness test for community-residing older adults. *Journal of Aging and Physical Activity, 7*, 129–161.

Rikli, R. E., & Jones, C. J. (1999). Functional fitness normative scores for community-residing older adults, ages 60–94. *Journal of Aging and Physical Activity, 7*, 162–182.

Rikli, R. E., & Jones, C. J. (2001). *Senior fitness test manual.* Champaign, IL: Human Kinetics.

■ SIT-UPS FOR ENDURANCE TEST

Objective: Measure abdominal muscle endurance

Age Range: Child to adult

Equipment Needed:

1. Exercise mat(s)
2. Stopwatch

Additional Personnel Needed: Test partner

Setup: Three sit-up variations are acceptable. The one the test performer chooses is dependent on his or her personal preference. For the most reliable and valid test results, the test administrator should document the sit-up variation and ensure that the test performer uses the same variation on subsequent tests.

Variation 1: The test performer's arms are crossed on the chest with the hands on opposite shoulders. The test performer begins with the mid-back contacting the mat (**Figure 4-22**). During the sit-up, the test performer touches the thigh with the arms still on the chest (**Figure 4-23**).

Variation 2: The test performer's hands are interlocked behind the neck. The test performer begins with the entire back touching the mat (**Figure 4-24**). During the sit-up, the test performer touches the elbows to the knees (**Figure 4-25**).

Variation 3: The test performer's hands are cupped behind the ears. The test performer begins with the entire back touching the mat (**Figure 4-26**). During the sit-up, the test performer touches the elbows to the knees (**Figure 4-27**).

No matter which sit-up variation is chosen, the test performer's heels are placed 12 to 18 inches (30 to 45 centimeters) from the buttocks, and a test partner stabilizes the test performer's feet on the mat.

Administration and Directions:

1. On the test administrator's "go" command, the test performer completes as many sit-ups as possible (while maintaining the chosen sit-up variation) for 1 minute.

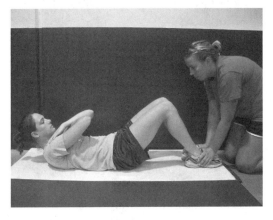

Figure 4-22   Variation 1: Sit-Ups for Endurance Test Setup

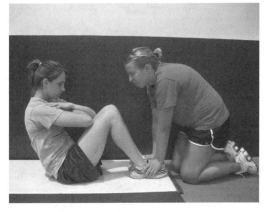

Figure 4-23   Variation 1: Sit-Ups for Endurance Test Administration

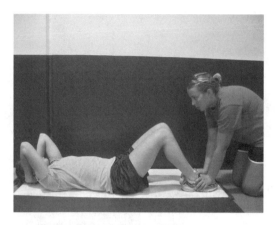

Figure 4-24 Variation 2: Sit-Ups for Endurance Test Setup

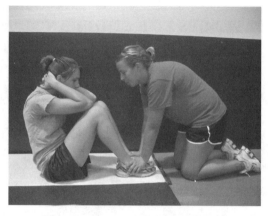

Figure 4-25 Variation 2: Sit-Ups for Endurance Test Administration

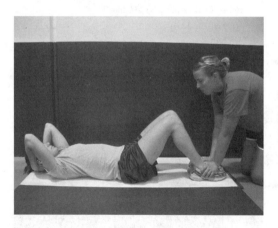

Figure 4-26 Variation 3: Sit-Ups for Endurance Test Administration

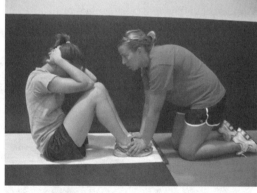

Figure 4-27 Variation 3: Sit-Ups for Endurance Test Administration

2. The test performer should be encouraged to perform the sit-ups at a comfortable, self-determined, and constant pace.
3. One trial is performed.

Scoring:

1. Each properly completed sit-up is counted as 1.

2. The total number of proper sit-ups completed in 1 minute is recorded as the final score. Some test protocols may have a test length of 2 minutes.

Checklist: The test performer must

1. Maintain the chosen sit-up variation for the duration of the test

2. Touch the proper part of the arms to the thighs (dependent upon the arm variation)
3. Touch the back to the mat (dependent upon the arm variation)
4. Not raise the buttocks off the ground at the beginning of the sit-up
5. Keep the feet stabilized on the floor 12 to 18 inches (30 to 45 centimeters) away from the buttocks

References

American Association for Health, Physical Education, Recreation, and Dance. (1976). *AAHPER youth fitness test manual.* Washington, DC: AAHPERD.

American Association for Health, Physical Education, Recreation, and Dance. (1980). *Lifetime health related physical fitness.* Reston, VA: AAHPERD.

Barnekow-Bergkvist, M., Hedberg, G., Janlert, U., & Jansson, E. (1996). Development of muscular endurance and strength from adolescence to adulthood and level of physical capacity in men and women at the age of 34 years. *Scandinavian Journal of Medicine and Science in Sports, 6,* 145–155.

Brodie, D. A. (1996). *A reference manual for human performance measurement in the field of physical education and sports sciences.* Lewiston, NY: Edwin Mellen Press.

Chung, P. K., & Yuen, C. K. (1999). Criterion-related validity of sit-and-reach tests in university men in Hong Kong. *Perceptual and Motor Skills, 88,* 204–316.

Huang, Y. C., & Malina, R. M. (2007). BMI and health-related physical fitness in Taiwanese youth 9–18 years. *Medicine and Science in Sports and Exercise, 39*(4), 701–708.

Jackson, A. W., Morrow, J. R., Brill, P. A., Kohl, H. W., Gordon, N. F., & Blair, S.N. (1998). Relations of sit-up and sit-and-reach tests to low back pain in adults. *Journal of Orthopedic and Sports Physical Therapy, 27*(1), 22–26.

Johnson, B. L., & Nelson, J. K. (1986). *Practical measurements for evaluation in physical education* (4th ed.). New York: MacMillan.

Meir, R., Newton, R., Curtis, E., Fardell, M., & Butler, B. (2001). Physical fitness qualities of professional rugby league football players: Determination of positional differences. *Journal of Strength and Conditioning Research, 15*(4), 450–458.

Miller, D. K. (2006). *Measurement by the physical educator: Why and how* (5th ed.). New York: McGraw-Hill.

Parfrey, K. C., Docherty, D., Workman, R. C., & Behm, D. G. (2008). The effects of different sit- and curl-up positions on activation of abdominal and hip flexor musculature. *Applied Physiology, Nutrition, and Metabolism, 33,* 888–895.

Roetert, E. P., Brown, S. W., Piorkowski, P. A., & Woods, R. B. (1996). Fitness comparisons among three different levels of elite tennis players. *Journal of Strength and Conditioning Research, 10*(3), 139–143.

Roetert, E. P, Piorkowski, P. A., Woods, R. B., & Brown, S. W. (1995). Establishing percentiles for junior tennis players based on physical fitness testing results. *Clinics in Sports Medicine, 14*(1), 1–21.

Safrit, M. J. (1995). *Complete guide to youth fitness testing.* Champaign, IL: Human Kinetics.

Semenick, D. (1981). Conditioning program: Testing and evaluation. *National Strength and Conditioning Association Journal, 3*(2): 8–9.

Semenick, D., Connors, J., Carter, M., Harman, E., et al. (1992). Test and measurement: Rationale, protocols, testing/reporting forms and instructions for wrestling. *National Strength and Conditioning Association Journal, 14*(3), 54–59.

■ ABDOMINAL CURL FOR ENDURANCE TEST

Also Known as: YMCA Half Sit-Up Test or Curl-Up Test

Objective: Measure abdominal muscle endurance

Age Range: Child to adult

Equipment Needed:

1. Stopwatch
2. Exercise mat(s)
2. Athletic tape

Additional Personnel Needed: None

Setup:

1. A strip of tape 3 inches (7.6 centimeters) wide is placed on the exercise mat. Commercial products are available in place of utilizing tape.
2. The test performer assumes a supine position on the exercise mat with the fingertips at the edge of the strip of tape with the arms straight at the sides (**Figure 4-28**).
3. The test performer's feet should be flat on the exercise mat with the heels as close to the hips as possible. The knees should be bent to approximately 140°.

4. The test performer may practice the protocol (described below) to become accustomed to the motion.

Administration and Directions:

1. On the test administrator's "go" command, the test performer curls forward until the fingertips move forward to the opposite end of the line and curls backward until the scapulas touch the exercise mat (**Figure 4-29**).
2. The test performer's scapulas must lift from the exercise mat during each curl, but the lower back should stay in contact with the exercise mat.
3. The test performer's feet should not lift off the exercise mat, and the feet should not be held.
4. The test performer should move in a slow and controlled self-directed pace.
5. The test performer completes as many abdominal curls as possible in 1 minute.
6. One trial is performed.

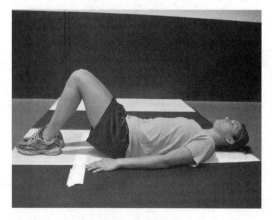

Figure 4-28 Abdominal Curl for Endurance Test Setup

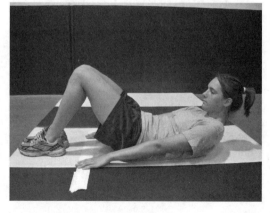

Figure 4-29 Abdominal Curl for Endurance Test Administration

Scoring:

1. Each properly completed curl-up is counted as 1.
2. The total number of proper curl-ups completed in 1 minute is recorded as the final score.

Checklist: The test performer must

1. Maintain the correct position during the test
2. Lift the scapulas from the exercise mat and return them to the exercise mat on each attempt
3. Not lift the lower back from the exercise mat during the test
4. Not have the feet held

References

Barnekow-Bergkvist, M., Hedberg, G., Janlert, U., & Jansson, E. (1996). Development of muscular endurance and strength from adolescence to adulthood and level of physical capacity in men and women at the age of 34 years. *Scandinavian Journal of Medicine and Science in Sports, 6,* 145–155.

Getchell, B., Mikesky, A. E., & Mikesky, K. N. (1998). *Physical fitness: A way of life* (5th ed.). Boston: Allyn and Bacon.

Golding, L. A. (2000). *YMCA fitness testing and assessment manual* (4th ed.). Champaign, IL: Human Kinetics.

Golding, L. A., Sinning, W. E., & Myers, C. R. (2000). *Y's way to physical fitness* Champaign, IL: Human Kinetics.

Heyward, V. H. (2006). *Advanced fitness assessment and exercise prescription* (5th ed.). Champaign, IL: Human Kinetics.

Johnson, B. L., & Nelson, J. K. (1986). *Practical measurements for evaluation in physical education* (4th ed.). New York: MacMillan.

Macfarlane, P. (1993). Out with the sit-up, in with the curl-p. *Journal of Physical Education, Recreation, and Dance, 64*(6), 62.

Meredith, M. D., & Welk, C. J. *FITNESSGRAM®/ ACTIVITYGRAM® test administration manual* (4th ed.). Champaign, IL: Human Kinetics.

Parfrey, K. C., Docherty, D., Workman, R. C., & Behm, D. G. (2008). The effects of different sit- and curl-up positions on activation of abdominal and hip flexor musculature. *Applied Physiology, Nutrition, and Metabolism, 33,* 888–895.

Payne, N,, Gledhill, N., Katzmarzyk, P. T., & Jamnik, V. (2000). Health-related fitness, physical activity, and history of back pain. *Canadian Journal of Applied Physiology, 25*(4), 236–249.

Safrit, M. J. (1995). *Complete guide to youth fitness testing.* Champaign, IL: Human Kinetics.

Tritschler, K. (2000). *Barrow & McGee's practical measurement and assessment* (5th ed.). Philadelphia: Lippincott Williams & Wilkins.

■ STATIC LEG ENDURANCE TEST

Also Known as: Wall Sit Test or Phantom Chair Test

Objective: Measure static thigh and lower-extremity muscle endurance

Age Range: Child to adult

Equipment Needed:

1. Stopwatch
2. Wall
3. Floor that is not excessively slick

Additional Personnel Needed: None

Setup:

1. The test performer places the back flat against the wall with the feet flat on the floor. The toes are pointed straight out, away from the wall (**Figure 4-30**).
2. The test performer may wear shoes.

Administration and Directions:

1. On the test performer's "go" command, the test performer slides the back down the wall until the knees are at a 90° angle. The toes should remain pointing straight out, away from the wall, with the feet flat on the floor. The arms should hang straight down, not touching the wall or the test performer's body (**Figure 4-31**).

2. The test performer maintains this position until exhaustion.
3. One trial is performed.

Scoring:

1. Once the test performer obtains the proper test position, the test administrator starts timing the trial.
2. The test administrator stops timing the test when the test performer breaks the proper position.
3. The time the test performer holds the proper test position is recorded as the final score.

Checklist: The test performer must

1. Keep the feet flat on the ground, with the toes pointing straight out, away from the wall

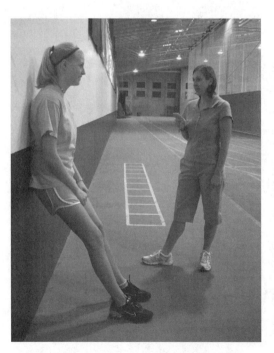

Figure 4-30 Static Leg Endurance Test Setup

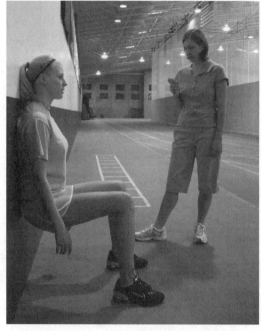

Figure 4-31 Static Leg Endurance Test Administration

2. Keep the arms hanging straight down and not touch the wall or the body with the hands
3. Keep the knees at a 90° angle and not reset the body once the proper position is broken

References

Miller, D. K. (2006). *Measurement by the physical educator: Why and how* (5th ed.). New York: McGraw-Hill.

Safrit, M. J. (1995). *Complete guide to youth fitness testing.* Champaign, IL: Human Kinetics.

■ 30-SECOND CHAIR STAND TEST

Objective: Measure lower-body muscular endurance

Age Range: 60 to 90+

Equipment Needed:

1. Stopwatch
2. Straight back or folding chair with a seat height of approximately 17 inches (43 centimeters) without arm rests
3. Wall
4. Flat floor with good traction

Additional Personnel Needed: None

Setup:

1. The chair is securely placed against the wall.
2. The test performer sits in the middle of the chair, with the back straight, feet flat on the floor, and arms crossed and held against the chest (**Figure 4-32**).
3. The test performer is allowed to practice the proper standing procedure (described below) for one to three repetitions.

Administration and Directions:

1. On the test administrators "go" command, the test performer rises from the chair to a full standing position (knees straight) while keeping the arms in the proper position (**Figure 4-33**).

2. Once the test performer achieves the full standing position, he or she sits back down in the chair in the starting position.

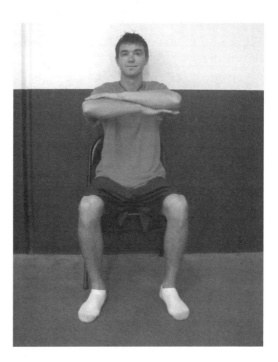

Figure 4-32 30-Second Chair Stand Test Setup

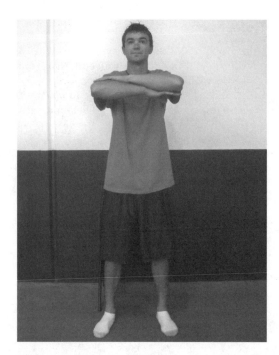

Figure 4-33 30-Second Chair Stand Test Administration

3. The test performer repeats this protocol continuously at a comfortable, self-determined, and constant pace for 30 seconds.
4. One trial is performed.

Scoring:

1. The total number of proper chair stands performed in 30 seconds is recorded as the final score.
2. If a test performer is more than halfway standing when the time expires, it is considered a complete stand.

Checklist: The test performer must

1. Extend the knees fully when standing
2. Not use the hands or arms for assistance in the standing or sitting motions
3. Completely sit on the chair between standing attempts
4. Not move faster then he or she feels comfortable

References

Cavani, V., Mier, C. M., Musto, A. A., & Tummers, N. (2002). Effects of a 6-week resistance-training program on functional fitness of older adults. *Journal of Aging and Physical Activity, 10,* 443–452.

Jones, C. J., Rikli, R. E., & Beam, W. C. (1999). A 30-s chair-stand test as a measure of lower body strength in community-residing older adults. *Research Quarterly for Exercise and Sports, 70*(2), 113–119.

Morrow, J. R., Jackson, A. W., Disch, J. G., & Mood, D. P. (2005). *Measurement and evaluation in human performance* (3rd ed.). Champaign, IL: Human Kinetics.

Rikli, R. E., & Jones, C. J. (1999). Development and validation of a functional fitness test for community-residing older adults. *Journal of Aging and Physical Activity, 7,* 129–161.

Rikli, R. E., & Jones, C. J. (1999). Functional fitness normative scores for community-residing older adults, ages 60–94. *Journal of Aging and Physical Activity, 7,* 162–182.

Rikli, R. E., & Jones, C. J. (2001). *Senior fitness test manual.* Champaign, IL: Human Kinetics.

■ BACK EXTENSOR ENDURANCE TEST

Objective: Measure static muscular endurance of the back extensor musculature

Age Range: Adult

Equipment Needed:

1. Sturdy and stable padded table
2. Straps
3. Stopwatch

Additional Personnel Needed: One or two test assistants

Setup:

1. The test performer lies prone on the padded table with the upper body hanging over the edge (**Figure 4-34**).
2. The test performer's buttocks and legs are secured to the table by the straps and/or the test assistant(s).
3. The test performer crosses the arms tight against the chest or behind the head.

Administration and Directions:

1. On the test administrator's "go" command, the test performer raises the body until he or she is horizontal with the table (**Figure 4-35**).
2. The test performer then holds that position until exhaustion, or a maximum of 240 seconds (4 minutes).
3. The test administrator or test assistant(s) may be required to assist the test performer lower the body once the trial is concluded.
4. One trial is performed.

Scoring:

1. The test administrator begins timing the trial when the test performer obtains the proper test position and stops timing the trial when the test performer no longer maintains the proper test position.
2. The number of seconds the test performer holds the proper test position is recorded as the final score.

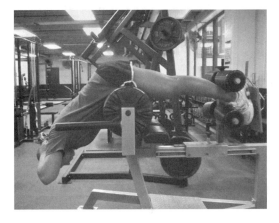

Figure 4-34 Back Extensor Endurance Test Setup

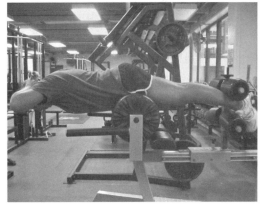

Figure 4-35 Back Extensor Endurance Test Administration

Checklist: The test performer must

1. Be secured to the table
2. Be horizontal with the table while the test is being timed
3. Keep the arms securely held to the chest or behind the head during the trial

References

Barnekow-Bergkvist, M., Hedberg, G., Janlert, U., & Jansson, E. (1996). Development of muscular endurance and strength from adolescence to adulthood and level of physical capacity in men and women at the age of 34 years. *Scandinavian Journal of Medicine and Science in Sports, 6,* 145–155.

Biering-Sorensen, F. (1984). Physical measurements as risk indicators of low-back trouble over a one-year period. *Spine, 9*(2), 106–119.

Hansen, J. W. (1964). Postoperative management in lumbar disc protrusions. *Acta Orthopedica Scandinavica, Suppl,* 71, 1–47.

Jorgensen, K., & Nicholaisen, T. (1986). Two methods for determining trunk extensor endurance. *European Journal of Applied Physiology, 55,* 639–644.

McGill, S. M., Childs, A., & Liebenson, C. (1999). Endurance times for low back stabilization exercises: Clinical targets for testing and training from a normal database. *Archives of Physical Medicine and Rehabilitation, 80,* 941–944.

Nesser, T. W., Huxel, K. C., Tincher, J. L., & Okada, T. (2008). The relationship between core stability and performance in division I football players. *Journal of Strength and Conditioning Research, 22*(6), 1750–1754.

Payne, N., Gledhill, N., Katzmarzyk, P. T., & Jamnik, V. (2000). Health-related fitness, physical activity, and history of back pain. *Canadian Journal of Applied Physiology, 25*(4), 236–249.

Suni, J. H., Miilunpalo, S. I., Asikainen, T. M., et al. (1998). Safety and feasibility of a health-related fitness test battery for adults. *Physical Therapy, 78*(2), 134–148: 1998.

Suni, J. H., Oja, P., Miilunpalo, S. I., Pasanen, M. E., Vuori, I. M., & Bos, K. (1998). Health-related fitness test battery for adults: Associations with perceived health, mobility, and back function and symptoms. *Archives of Physical Medicine and Rehabilitation, 79,* 559–569.

Tritschler, K. (2000). *Barrow & McGee's practical measurement and assessment* (5th ed.). Philadelphia: Lippincott Williams & Wilkins.

CHAPTER

5

Balance Testing

Balance is the body's ability to maintain equilibrium against the forces of gravity. Balance is made up of the kinesthetic sense of the muscles, the inner ear, and visual perception of the environment. Balance is generally evaluated while standing on, jumping to, or landing on one or both legs. There are two types of balance that are essential to successful movement: static balance and dynamic balance. Static balance is the body's ability to maintain equilibrium while stationary. Dynamic balance is the body's ability to maintain equilibrium while in motion or moving the body or body parts to another position.

The test administrator should ensure that the test performer has reasonable balance before the balance is tested. Any acute or chronic injuries to, or involving, the lower extremities or the brain may adversely affect balance. Testing an individual with limited balance may result in injury. If the test administrator is unsure of a test performer's balancing ability, a preliminary one-leg balance test should be conducted in which the test performer can brace him- or herself (against either a wall or the test administrator). Shoes provide external stability to the foot and ankle during balance testing. So, unless otherwise noted or required, test performers should remove their footwear during balance testing. To increase the difficulty of any balance test, the test performer may close the eyes (and/or tilt the head back) or balance on an unstable surface (i.e., foam). Balance tests generally do not result in fatigue, but they may be negatively influenced by previous physical fitness tests. For best results, balance tests should not be conducted immediately after lower-body strength, agility, speed, local muscular endurance, or cardiovascular physical fitness tests.

■ STORK STAND TEST

Objective: Measure static balance

Age Range: 10 to adult

Equipment Needed:

1. Stopwatch
2. Open, solid flat surface

Additional Personnel Needed: None

Setup:

1. The test performer stands and places the hands on the hips.
2. The test performer then stands on the dominant leg (the leg they would prefer to kick a ball with) and places the non-dominant foot against the inside of the supporting knee while keeping the hands on the hips (**Figure 5-1**).

3. The test administrator may want to stand profile to the test performer for the best view of the test performer's heel.

Administration and Directions:

1. On the test administrator's "go" command, the test performer goes up on the ball of the dominant foot (the heel comes off the ground) (**Figure 5-2**).
2. The test performer maintains the balance position as long as possible.
3. The test administrator can conduct this test for each foot, testing one foot at a time.
4. Three trials are performed.

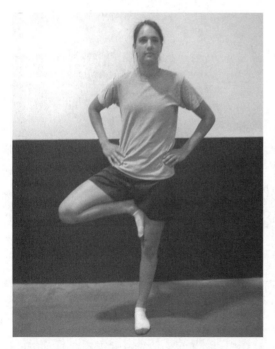

Figure 5-1   Stork Stand Test Setup

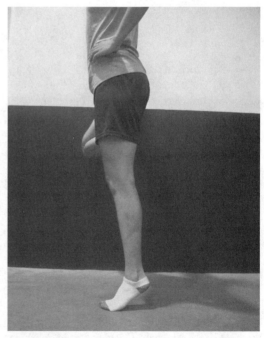

Figure 5-2   Stork Stand Test Administration

Scoring:

1. The test administrator starts timing when the test performer is in the proper test position.
2. The test administrator stops timing when the test performer:
   a. No longer maintains balance on the *ball* of the dominant foot (when the heel touches the ground).
   b. No longer maintains the hands on the hips.
   c. Moves the balance foot from its original position.
   d. No longer maintains the non-dominant leg in its original position.
3. There is no time limit on this test.
4. The longest time is recorded as the final score. The test administrator should document the leg the test performer balanced on or the best time for each foot.

Checklist: The test performer must

1. Remove his or her shoes
2. Be in the proper position before the "go" command is given

References

Barnekow-Bergkvist, M., Hedberg, G., Janlert, U., & Jansson, E. (1996). Development of muscular endurance and strength from adolescence to adulthood and level of physical capacity in men and women at the age of 34 years. *Scandinavian Journal of Medicine, Science, and Sports, 6*, 145–155.

Brodie, D. A. (1996). *A reference manual for human performance measurement in the field of physical education and sports sciences.* Lewiston, NY: Edwin Mellen Press.

Greene, J. J., McGuine, T. A., Leverson, G., & Best, T. M. (1998). Anthropometric and performance measures for high school basketball players. *Journal of Athletic Training, 33*(3), 229–232.

Johnson, B. L., & Nelson, J. K. (1986). *Practical measurements for evaluation in physical education* (4th ed.). New York: MacMillan.

Miller, D. K. (2006). *Measurement by the physical educator: Why and how* (5th ed.). New York: McGraw-Hill.

Ribadi, H., Rider, R. A., & Toole, T. (1987). A comparison of static and dynamic balance in congenitally blind, sighted, and sighted blindfolded adolescents. *Adapted Physical Activity Quarterly, 4*, 220–225.

Rinne, M. B., Pasanen, M. E., Miilunpalo, S. I., & Oja, P. (2001). Test-retest reproducibility and inter-rater reliability of a motor skill test battery for adults. *International Journal of Sports Medicine, 22*, 192–200.

Roth, A. E., Miller, M. G., Ricard, M., Ritenour, D., & Chapman, B. L. (2006). Comparisons of static and dynamic balance following training in aquatic and land environments. *Journal of Sport Rehabilitation, 15*, 299–311.

Suni, J. H., Miilunpalo, S. I., Asikainen, T. M., et al. (1998). Safety and feasibility of a health-related fitness test battery for adults. *Physical Therapy, 78*(2), 134–148.

Suni, J. H., Oja, P., Miilunpalo, S. I., Pasanen, M. E., Vuori, I. M., & Bos, K. (1998). Health-related fitness test battery for adults: Associations with perceived health, mobility, and back function and symptoms. *Archives of Physical Medicine and Rehabilitation, 79*, 559–569.

Tritschler, K. (2000). *Barrow & McGee's practical measurement and assessment* (5th ed.). Philadelphia: Lippincott Williams & Wilkins.

■ BASS STICK TEST (LENGTHWISE)

Objective: Measure static balance

Age Range: 10 to adult

Equipment Needed:

1. Stopwatch
2. Athletic tape
3. 1- by 1- by 12-inch (2.5- by 2.5- by 30-centimeter) stick
4. Open, solid flat surface

Additional Personnel Needed: None

Setup:

1. The stick is secured to the floor using athletic tape.
2. The test performer places one foot lengthwise on the stick (the ball and heel of the foot are both in contact with the stick) (**Figure 5-3**).

Administration and Directions:

1. On the test administrator's "go" command, the test performer raises the heel of the test foot off the stick and lifts the opposite foot from the floor (**Figure 5-4**).
2. The test performer maintains the balance position as long as possible.
3. Three trials are performed for each foot.

Scoring:

1. If a test performer loses his or her balance in the first 3 seconds of a trial, the trial is stopped, considered invalid, and restarted.
2. The test administrator starts timing when the test performer is in the proper test position.

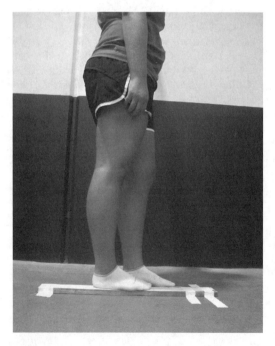

Figure 5-3 Bass Stick Test (Lengthwise) Setup

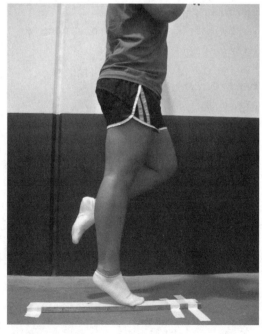

Figure 5-4 Bass Stick Test (Lengthwise) Administration

3. The test administrator stops timing when the test performer
   a. No longer maintains balance with the ball of the balance foot (when the heel touches the stick)
   b. Moves the balance foot from its original position
   c. Touches the ground with the non-balance foot
4. The best time (on each foot) is recorded as the final score.

Checklist: The test performer must

1. Remove his or her shoes
2. Place the foot on the center of the stick
3. Go up on the toes

References

Bass, R. I. (1939). An analysis of the components of tests of semicircular canal function and of static and dynamic balance. *Research Quarterly of the American Association for Health, Physical Education, and Recreation, 10*, 33–52.

Clark, J. E., & Watkins, D. L. (1984). Static balance in young children. *Child Development, 55*, 854–857.

DeOreo, K. D., & Wade, M. G. (1971). Dynamic and static balancing ability of pre-school children. *Journal of Motor Behavior, 3*(4), 326–335.

Johnson, B. L., & Nelson, J. K. (1986). *Practical measurements for evaluation in physical education* (4th ed.). New York: MacMillan.

Miller, D. K. (2006). *Measurement by the physical educator: Why and how* (5th ed.). New York: McGraw-Hill.

Rinne, M. B., Pasanen, M. E., Miilunpalo, S. I., & Oja, P. (2001). Test-retest reproducibility and inter-rater reliability of a motor skill test battery for adults. *International Journal of Sports Medicine, 22*, 192–200.

Sanborn, C., & Wyrick, W. (1969). Prediction of olympic balance beam performance from standardized and modified test of balance. *Research Quarterly, 40*(1), 174–184.

■ BASS STICK TEST (CROSSWISE)

Objective: Measure static balance

Age Range: 10 to adult

Equipment Needed:

1. Stopwatch
2. Athletic tape
3. 1- by 1- by 12-inch (2.5- by 2.5- by 30-centimeter) stick
4. Open, solid flat surface

Additional Personnel Needed: None

Setup:

1. The stick is secured to the floor using athletic tape.

2. The test performer places one foot crosswise on the stick (the ball of the foot is touching the stick, but the heel is in contact with the ground) (**Figure 5-5**).

Administration and Directions:

1. On the test administrator's "go" command, the test performer raises the heel of the test foot off the ground, and lifts the non-balance foot from the floor (**Figure 5-6**).
2. The test performer maintains the balance position as long as possible.
3. Three trials are performed on each foot.

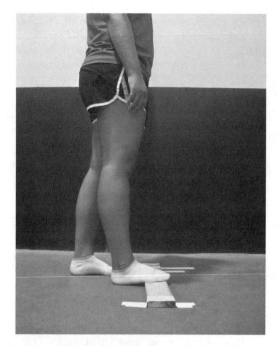

Figure 5-5   Bass Stick Test (Crosswise) Setup

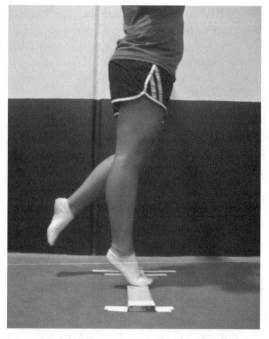

Figure 5-6   Bass Stick Test (Crosswise) Administration

Scoring:

1. If a test performer loses his or her balance in the first 3 seconds of a trial, the trial is stopped, considered invalid, and restarted.
2. The test administrator starts timing when the test performer is in the proper test position.
3. The test administrator stops timing when the test performer
   a. No longer maintains balance with the ball of the balance foot (when the heel touches the ground)
   b. Moves the balance foot from its original position
   c. Touches the ground with the non-balance foot
4. The best time (on each foot) is recorded as the final score.

Checklist: The test performer must

1. Remove his or her shoes
2. Place the ball of the foot on the center of the stick
3. Go up on the toes

References

Bass, R. I. (1939). An analysis of the components of tests of semicircular canal function and of static and dynamic balance. *Research Quarterly of the American Association for Health, Physical Education, and Recreation, 10,* 33–52.

Clark, J. E., & Watkins, D. L. (1984). Static balance in young children. *Child Development, 55,* 854–857.

DeOreo, K. D., & Wade, M. G. (1971). Dynamic and static balancing ability of pre-school children. *Journal of Motor Behavior, 3*(4), 326–335.

Johnson, B. L., & Nelson, J. K. (1986). *Practical measurements for evaluation in physical education* (4th ed.). New York: MacMillan.

Miller, D. K. (2006). *Measurement by the physical educator: Why and how* (5th ed.). New York: McGraw-Hill.

Rinne, M. B., Pasanen, M. E., Miilunpalo, S. I., & Oja, P. (2001). Test-retest reproducibility and inter-rater reliability of a motor skill test battery for adults. *International Journal of Sports Medicine, 22*, 192–200.

■ TANDEM STANCE TEST

Objective: Measure static balance

Age Range: Child to 60+

Equipment Needed:

1. Stopwatch
2. Open, solid flat surface

Additional Personnel Needed: None

Setup: The test performer stands.

Administration and Directions:

1. On the test administrator's "go" command, the test performer places the heel of one foot directly in front of the toes of the other foot. The test performer puts the foot of his or her choice forward (**Figure 5-7**).
2. The test performer holds that position as long as possible without taking a step.
3. Up to three trials are performed.

Scoring:

1. The test administrator starts timing when the test performer is in the proper test position and stops timing when the test performer moves from the proper test position.

2. The best time is recorded as the final score.

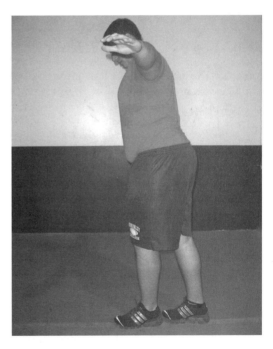

Figure 5-7 Tandem Stance Test Administration

3. Individuals who cannot hold the test position for at least 10 seconds are at a higher risk of falls.

Checklist: The test performer must

1. Be wearing appropriate footwear
2. Not hold onto an object during the test
3. Have reasonable balance before performing this test

References

Lark, S. D., & Pasupuleti, S. (2009). Validity of a functional dynamic walking test for the elderly.

Archives of Physical Medicine and Rehabilitation, 90, 470–474.

Roth, A. E., Miller, M. G., Ricard, M., Ritenour, D., & Chapman, B. L. (2006). Comparisons of static and dynamic balance following training in aquatic and land environments. *Journal of Sport Rehabilitation, 15,* 299–311.

Shubert, T. E., Schrodt, L. A., Mercer, V. S., Busby-Whitehead, J., & Giuliani, C. A. (2006). Are scores on balance screening tests associated with mobility in older adults? *Journal of Geriatric Physical Therapy, 29*(1), 33–39.

■ BALANCE BEAM WALK TEST

Objective: Measure dynamic balance while walking on a narrow area

Age Range: 9 to college age

Equipment Needed:

1. Stopwatch
2. Regulation balance beam, 4 inches (10 centimeters) wide and 16 feet (4.9 meters) long
3. A taped or permanent line of the same width and length on a flat, solid surface is acceptable if a balance beam is not available.

Additional Personnel Needed: Test assistant

Setup:

1. A standard balance beam is adjusted so that the test performer is elevated off the ground.

2. The test performer stands on one end of the balance beam. A test assistant may be needed to assist the test performer onto the balance beam.

Administration and Directions:

1. On the test administrator's "go" command, the test performer walks to the opposite end of the balance beam (**Figure 5-8**).
2. The test performer should complete this test at a comfortable, self-directed, and constant pace.
3. Once the test performer reaches the opposite end of the balance beam, he or she pauses for 5 seconds before turning around and walking back to the starting position.
4. Three trials may be performed.

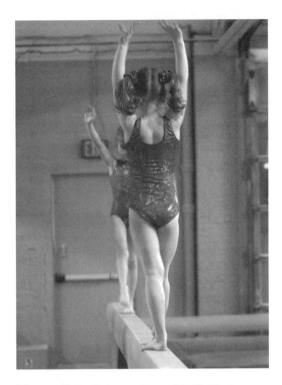

Figure 5-8   Balance Beam Walk Test
Administration

Scoring: The final score may be recorded as

1. The time it takes the test performer to complete this test *or*
2. Pass/fail (time does not matter)

Checklist: The test performer must

1. Be barefoot
2. Be properly balanced before beginning the test

3. Pause for 5 seconds before turning around and returning to the starting position

References

DeOreo, K. D., & Wade, M. G. (1971). Dynamic and static balancing ability of pre-school children. *Journal of Motor Behavior, 3*(4), 326–335.

Espenschade, A., Dable, R. A., & Schoendube, R. (1953). Dynamic balance in adolescent boys. *Research Quarterly of the American Association for Health, Physical Education, and Recreation, 24,* 270–275.

Miller, D. K. (2006). *Measurement by the physical educator: Why and how* (5th ed.). New York: McGraw-Hill.

Punakallio, A. (2004). Trial-to-trial reproducibility and test-retest stability of two dynamic balance tests among male firefighters. *International Journal of Sports Medicine, 25,* 163–169.

Seashore, H. G. (1947). The development of a beam-walking test and its use in measuring development of balance in children. *Research Quarterly of the American Association for Health, Physical Education, and Recreation, 18,* 246–259.

Tsigilis, N., Zachopoulou, E., & Mavridis, T. H. (2001). Evaluation of the specificity of selected dynamic balance tests. *Perceptual and Motor Skills, 92,* 827–833.

■ TANDEM WALKING TEST

Objective: Measure dynamic balance while walking on a narrow area

Age Range: Child to adult

Equipment Needed:

1. Stopwatch
2. Open, solid flat surface
3. Tape measure
4. Tape (or a permanent narrow solid line)

Additional Personnel Needed: None

Setup:

1. The test administrator locates or creates a solid line that is 6 meters (6.5 yards) long and approximately 2.5 centimeters (1 inch) wide.
2. The test performer stands on one end of the line with the heel of one foot directly touching the toes of the opposite foot in a heel-to-toe position.
3. The test performer may practice the protocol (described below) to become accustomed to the movement pattern.

Administration and Directions:

1. On the test administrator's "go" command, the test performer walks along the straight line by placing one foot in front of the other; the heel of the front foot is touching the toes of the trailing foot. The test performer may begin this test with either foot forward (**Figure 5-9**).
2. The test performer walks to the opposite end of the line.

3. The test performer should complete this test at a comfortable, self-directed, and constant pace.
4. If the test performer loses his or her balance or steps to the side, the trial is stopped, considered invalid, and restarted.
5. This test may be performed with the test performer walking forward or backward along the line.
6. Three complete trials are performed.

Scoring:

1. The test administrator records the time it takes the test performer to travel along the line.
2. The test administrator may choose to record the test performer's forward and backward walking times.
3. The fastest time is recorded as the final score.

Checklist: The test performer must

1. Be wearing appropriate footwear
2. Step with the heel of one foot touching the toes of the opposite foot
3. Walk in a straight line (i.e., the line directly under the test performer's feet should not be visible)

References

Lark, S. D., & Pasupuleti, S. (2009). Validity of a functional dynamic walking test for the elderly. *Archives of Physical Medicine and Rehabilitation, 90*, 470–474.

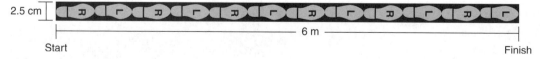

2.5 cm

6 m

Start

Finish

Figure 5-9 Tandem Walking Test Administration

Nelson, M. E., Fiatarone, M. A., Morganti, C. M., Trice, I., Greenberg, R. A., & Evans, W. J. (1994). Effects of high-intensity strength training on multiple risk factors for osteoporotic fractures. *Journal of the American Medical Association, 272*(24), 1909–1913.

Rinne, M. B., Pasanen, M. E., Miilunpalo, S. I., & Oja, P. (2001). Test-retest reproducibility and inter-rater reliability of a motor skill test battery for adults. *International Journal of Sports Medicine, 22*, 192–200.

Vereeck, L., Wuyts, F., Truijen, S., & Van de Heyning, P. (2008). Clinical assessment of balance: Normative data, and gender and age effects. *International Journal of Audiology, 47*, 67–75.

■ TIMED 360° TURN TEST

Objective: Measure dynamic balance

Age Range: Child to senior; this test is designed for seniors but can be used for other populations

Equipment Needed:

1. Stopwatch
2. Open, solid floor surface
3. Tape (or a permanent floor mark)

Additional Personnel Needed: None

Setup:

1. The test administrator creates a small X or utilizes a small permanent mark on the floor.
2. The test performer places one foot directly on the mark and faces the test administrator, with both feet pointing toward the test administrator.

Administration and Directions:

1. On the test administrator's "go" command, the test performer makes a complete circle (360°) by moving both feet as quickly as possible. The test performer may move in either direction (left or right) (**Figure 5-10**).

2. The foot placed on the X should not significantly deviate from the X during the trial.
3. The test performer ends the test facing the test administrator in the starting position.
4. Two trials are performed.

Scoring:

1. The test administrator begins timing when the test performer begins moving and stops timing when the test performer returns to the starting position.
2. The two trials are averaged and recorded as the final score.
3. A test performer who takes longer than 3.8 seconds to turn 360° may be at increased risk of falling.

Checklist: The test performer must

1. Have appropriate balance before beginning this test
2. Be wearing appropriate footwear
3. Begin and end each trial facing the same direction
4. Not significantly move the foot from the X during the test

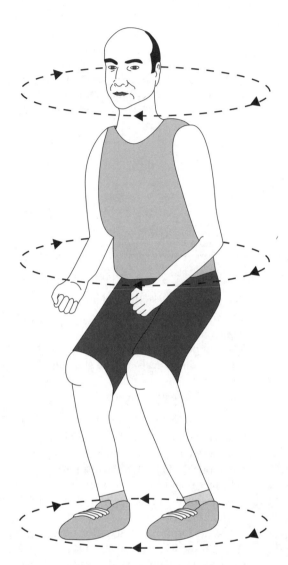

Figure 5-10 Timed 360° Turn Test Administration

Reference

Shubert, T. E., Schrodt, L. A., Mercer, V. S., Busby-Whitehead, J., & Giuliani, C. A. (2006). Are scores on balance screening tests associated with mobility in older adults? *Journal of Geriatric Physical Therapy, 29*(1), 33–39.

■ MODIFIED BASS DYNAMIC BALANCE TEST

Objective: Measure dynamic and static balance during movement and upon landing from a jump

Age Range: High school to college age

Equipment Needed:

1. Stopwatch
2. Open, solid flat surface
3. Tape measure

Additional Personnel Needed: Test assistant

Setup:

1. Eleven small pieces of tape approximately 1 inch by 1 inch (2.5 centimeters by 2.5 centimeters) are placed on the floor (**Figure 5-11**).
2. The test performer stands with the right foot placed on the starting tape mark.

Administration and Directions:

1. On the test administrator's "go" command, the test performer jumps to the next tape mark, landing on the ball of the left foot, and attempts to hold that position for 5 seconds (refer to Figure 5-11).
2. After 5 seconds, the test performer then jumps to the second tape mark, landing on the ball of the right foot, and attempts to hold that position for 5 seconds.
3. This process is continued throughout the remainder of the course.
4. The test administrator should count the 5-second balance phase aloud to the test performer.
5. One trial is performed.

Note: The ball of the foot must completely cover the tape mark; the test performer must land directly on the tape mark and maintain his or her balance on the tape mark for 5 seconds to successfully complete the test segment. At the conclusion of each 5-second balance attempt, the test performer immediately initiates the next jump.

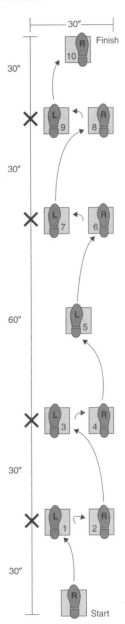

Figure 5-11 Modified Bass Dynamic Balance Test Course Setup and Administration

Scoring:

1. This test is scored in points according to the system described below.
   a. Five points are given if the test performer successfully lands on the designated tape mark correctly.
   b. One point is given for each second the test performer successfully maintains his or her balance (while on the ball of the foot) on each designated tape mark.
   c. The points the test performer earns on each jump and balance phase are added together.

The test performer should be penalized 5 points for any of the following landing errors.
   a. Failure to stop upon landing (taking an extra step)
   b. Touching the floor with any part of the body other than the *ball* of the landing foot (i.e., heel)
   c. Failure to correctly cover the designated tape mark with the *ball* of the foot

If a landing error occurs, the test performer should immediately regain the correct position and attempt the balance portion of the test.

If the test performer lands successfully, he or she should be penalized 1 point for either of the following balance errors.
   a. Touching the floor with any part of the body other than the *ball* of the landing foot (i.e., heel)
   b. Failing to maintain the balance position for 5 seconds

If a balance error occurs, the test performer should immediately regain the correct position and jump to the next tape mark.

2. A maximum of 10 points is possible for each tape mark.

3. A maximum of 100 points is possible for the entire test.
4. It is helpful for the test assistant to score the test. This may be done by having the test administrator and test assistant score separate portions of the test (i.e., landing or balance) or by having each score the entire test separately and compare their scores at the end.
5. The final point total is recorded as the final score.

Checklist: The test performer must

1. Have adequate balance before beginning this test
2. Land on the ball of their foot, completely covering the tape mark
3. Jump to the next tape mark once the test administrator counts to five
4. Understand the jumping pattern before beginning the test

References

Bass, R. I. (1939). An analysis of the components of tests of semicircular canal function and of static and dynamic balance. *Research Quarterly of the American Association for Health, Physical Education, and Recreation, 10,* 33–52.

Johnson, B. L., & Nelson, J. K. (1986). *Practical measurements for evaluation in physical education* (4th ed.). New York: MacMillan.

Miller, D. K. (2006). *Measurement by the physical educator: Why and how* (5th ed.). New York: McGraw-Hill.

Tsigilis, N., Zachopoulou, E., & Mavridis, T. H. (2001). Evaluation of the specificity of selected dynamic balance tests. *Perceptual and Motor Skills, 92,* 827–833.

■ MODIFIED SIDEWARD LEAP TEST

Objective: Measure dynamic and static balance during movement and upon landing from a leap.

Age Range: Middle school to college age

Equipment Needed:

1. Stopwatch
2. Open, solid flat surface
3. Tape measure
4. Floor tape
5. Small, light object (i.e., cork or thimble)

Additional Personnel Needed: Test assistant

Setup:

1. Three 1-inch (2.5-centimeter) square dots of tape are created in a straight line 18 inches (45 centimeters) apart on the floor (**Figure 5-12**).
2. Three or four Xs perpendicular to the center dot are created. These Xs should be 3 inches (7.6 centimeters) apart and start approximately 24 inches (61 centimeters) perpendicular to the center dot.
3. The test performer may practice the test protocol (described below) to become accustomed to the motion. The test administrator may need to create an X specific for an individual test performer if none of the standard Xs are deemed appropriate during practice or the test.
4. The small, light object is placed over dot B.
5. The test performer places the left foot on an X (balancing on that foot) with the right side toward dot A.

Administration and Directions:

1. On the test administrator's "go" command, the test performer leaps sideways with the objective of landing on the ball of the right foot directly on dot A (refer to Figure 5-12).
2. A leap is a motion in which both feet are off the ground simultaneously, but excessive effort should not be required to perform the action.

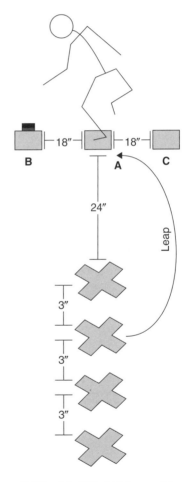

Figure 5-12 Modified Sideward Leap Test Setup and Administration

3. Once the test performer lands on the ball of the right foot, he or she immediately leans forward and attempts to knock the object off dot B without touching the floor with the hand or fingers.
4. Once the attempt to knock the object off dot B is completed (successfully or unsuccessfully), the test performer attempts to maintain balance on the ball of the right foot for 5 seconds. The test performer may maintain balance in either a flexed or an erect trunk position.
5. Once the test performer has held his or her balance for 5 seconds (or fails), the trial is complete and the course is reset.
6. Four trials are performed: two trials as described above and two trials of the reverse (the object is placed on dot C, with the test performer initially balancing on the ball of the right foot and jumping onto the ball of the left foot).

Scoring:

1. This test is scored in points, utilizing the system described below:
   a. The maximum number of points possible for each trial is 15.
   b. Five points are awarded for landing correctly on dot A.
   c. Five points are awarded for properly pushing the object off dot B or C.
   d. One point is awarded for each second the test performer successfully maintains balance on dot A after attempting to knock the object off dot B or C (up to 5 seconds).
2. The best score is recorded as the final score for each foot.

Checklist: The test performer must

1. Balance on one leg before leaping onto the other
2. Understand how to leap
3. Land on the ball of the foot
4. Attempt to maintain balance if the object is not successfully knocked off a dot

References

Miller, D. K. (2006). *Measurement by the physical educator: Why and how* (5th ed.). New York: McGraw-Hill.

Sanborn, C., & Wyrick, W. (1969). Prediction of Olympic balance beam performance from standardized and modified test of balance. *Research Quarterly, 40*(1), 174–184.

■ STAR EXCURSION BALANCE TEST (SEBT)

Objective: Quickly assess dynamic balance

Age Range: Child to adult

Equipment Needed:

1. Open, solid flat surface
2. Tape measure
3. Tape (preferably white)
4. Marking pen

Additional Personnel Needed: Test assistant

Setup:

1. Create four 8-feet (2.4-meter)-long strips of tape (**Figure 5-13**).
2. Two strips of tape are placed in the shape of a cross on the floor.

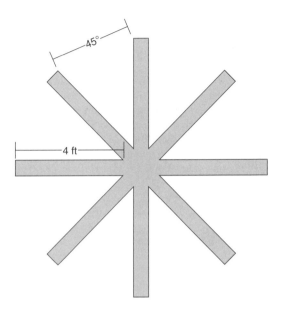

Figure 5-13 Star Excursion Balance Test Setup

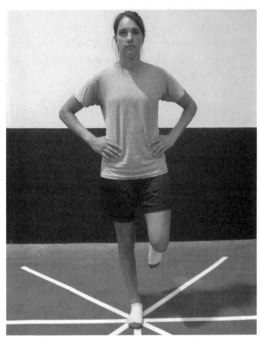

Figure 5-14 Star Excursion Balance Test Starting Position

3. The other two strips of tape are placed in the shape of a cross, offset on the first cross by 45°.
4. The final shape should be a star with eight lines 45° apart. It should be 4 feet (1.2 meters) from the center of the star to the end of each strip of tape.
5. The test performer places the test foot in the center of the star, with the foot facing directly forward along a taped line (**Figure 5-14**).

Administration and Directions:

1. On the test administrator's "go" command, the test performer balances on the test foot and reaches with the toe of the opposite foot (reach foot) along each strip of tape as far as possible (**Figure 5-15**).
2. The test performer touches the farthest point along the tape with either the toes or the forefoot only of the reach foot.

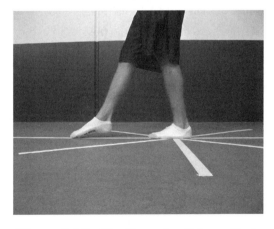

Figure 5-15 Star Excursion Balance Test Administration

3. The reach foot should not be used for support when it touches the floor.
4. The test performer maintains the reached position until the test assistant can mark the distance with the pen.
5. After the distance is marked, the test performer returns to the starting position before reaching along the next strip of tape. This process is completed for each of the eight directions.
6. The test performer then switches feet and performs the same protocol with the opposite foot.
7. One trial is performed on each foot.

Scoring:

1. The distance from the star's center to each mark is measured.
2. A mark does not count if the test performer
   a. Loses balance while reaching along the taped line
   b. Uses the reach foot for support when it touches the floor
3. The distance of the reach on each foot (in each direction) is recorded as the final score.

Checklist: The test performer must

1. Keep the balance foot in the star's center
2. Not use the reach foot for support

References

Bressel, E., Yonker, J. C., Kras, J., & Heath, E. M. (2007). Comparison of static and dynamic balance in female collegiate soccer, basketball, and gymnastic athletics. *Journal of Athletic Training, 42*(1), 42–46.

Brumitt, J. (2008). Assessing athletic balance with the star excursion balance test. *NSCA's Performance Training Journal, 7*(3), 6–7.

Earl, J. E., & Hertel, J. (2001). Lower-extremity muscle activation during the star excursion balance test. *Journal of Sport Rehabilitation, 10*, 93–104.

Gribble, P. A., & Hertel, J. (2003). Predictors for performance of dynamic postural control using the star excursion balance test. *Measurement in Physical Education and Exercise Science, 7*, 89–100.

Gribble, P. (2003). The star excursion balance test as a measurement tool. *Athletic Therapy Today, 8*(2), 46–47.

Gribble, P. A., Tucker, W. S., & White, P. A. (2007). Time-of-day influence on static and dynamic postural control. *Journal of Athletic Training, 42*(1), 35–41.

Hardy, L., Huxel, K., Brucker, J., & Nesser, T. (2008). Prophylactic Ankle Braces and Star Excursion Balance Measures in Health Volunteers. *Journal of Athletic Training, 43*(4), 347–351.

Hertel, J., Miller, S., & Denegar, C. (2000). Intratester and intertester reliability during the star excursion balance test. *Journal of Sport Rehabilitation, 9*, 104–116.

Herrington, L., Hatcher, J., Hatcher, A., & McNicholas, M. (2009). A comparison of star excursion balance test reach distances between ACL deficient patients and asymptomatic controls. *The Knee, 16*, 149–152.

Kinzey, S. J., & Armstrong, C. W. (1998). The reliability of the star-excursion test in assessing dynamic balance. *Journal of Orthopaedic and Sports Physical Therapy, 27*(5), 356–360.

Olmsted, L. C., Carcia, C. R., Hertel, J., & Shultz, S. J. (2002). Efficacy of the star excursion balance tests in detecting reach deficits in subjects with chronic ankle instability. *Journal of Athletic Training, 37*(4), 501–506.

CHAPTER

6

Strength Testing

Muscular strength is the body's (or body parts') ability to exert maximal effort, generally the amount of force a muscular group can produce for a single, maximum effort. Muscular strength tests are performed at slow speeds and require between 2 and 4 seconds to complete. Muscular strength tests can be recorded as either absolute or relative strength. *Absolute strength* is the total amount of weight the test performer can lift regardless of his or her body weight. *Relative strength* is the total amount of weight the test performer can lift in relationship to his or her body weight. To record a test performer's relative strength, first measure his or her body weight and then measure the amount of weight the test performer lifts during the test session. To calculate the relative strength, which can be recorded as a percent or a ratio, divide the weight lifted by the performer's body weight.

Muscular strength tests must be performed with proper technique for reliable and valid results as well as safety. The test administrator should ensure that the test performer can execute the strength test with proper technique at a lower intensity before additional weight is applied. If the test performer cannot maintain, or does not possess, proper technique at lower weight, additional weight should not be applied before the test performer's technique is developed. The test administrator should ensure that the test performer warms up properly by performing the strength test activity with lighter weights and gradually increasing weight until the test administrator can actually measure the test performer's maximal effort. Test administrators should educate the test performers about the Valsalva maneuver. The Valsalva maneuver is a process that increases abdominal rigidity and blood pressure, aiding in protecting the lower back from injury and assisting the individual to lift more weight. If the test administrator wants to prevent the occurrence of a Valsalva maneuver, he or she should ensure that the test performer exhales during the strenuous portion of the muscular strength test. Muscular strength tests should be performed before local muscular endurance and cardiovascular fitness tests.

■ HANDGRIP STRENGTH (DYNAMOMETER) TEST

Objective: Measure handgrip strength

Age Range: 5 to adult

Equipment Needed:

1. Handgrip dynamometer

Additional Personnel Needed: None

Setup:

1. The test performer stands erect and is given the handgrip dynamometer. The handgrip dynamometer should be set to 0.
2. The handgrip dynamometer should be adjusted to fit comfortably in the test performer's hand where the proximal interphalangeal (PIP) joints of the fingers should be under the handle (**Figure 6-1**).
3. The test performer holds the handgrip dynamometer at his or her side by the waist with the forearm parallel to the thigh. The elbow may be slightly flexed (**Figure 6-2**).

Administration and Directions:

1. On the test administrator's "go" command, the test performer squeezes the bar on the handgrip dynamometer as hard as possible.
2. The test performer should exhale while the handgrip dynamometer is squeezed.
3. Once the test performer has completed the trial, the test administrator records

the trial, resets the hand dynamometer to 0, and has the test performer conduct the same protocol on the opposite hand.

4. Three trials are performed for each hand.

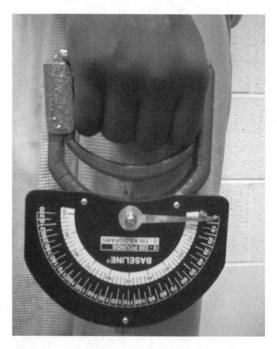

Figure 6-1   Handgrip Strength Test Hand Position

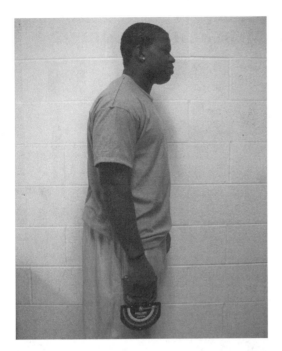

Figure 6-2 Handgrip Strength Test Setup

Scoring:

1. Each trial is recorded.
2. The highest trial for each hand is recorded as the final score.
3. Some scoring criteria may require adding the highest score from each hand into a single score.

Checklist: The test performer must

1. Be standing during each trial
2. Exhale during the trial
3. Allow the test administrator to see and record the score at the end of each trial

References

Barnekow-Bergkvist, M., Hedberg, G., Janlert, U., & Jansson, E. (1996). Development of muscular endurance and strength from adolescence to adulthood and level of physical capacity in men and women at the age of 34 years. *Scandinavian Journal of Medicine, Science, and Sports, 6,* 145–155.

Brodie, D. A. (1996). *A reference manual for human performance measurement in the field of physical education and sports sciences.* Lewiston, NY: Edwin Mellen Press.

Heyward, V. H. (2006). *Advanced fitness assessment and exercise prescription* (5th ed.). Champaign, IL: Human Kinetics.

Johnson, B. L., & Nelson, J. K. (1986). *Practical measurements for evaluation in physical education* (4th ed.). New York: MacMillan.

Keough, J. W. L., Weber, C. L., & Dalton, C. T. (2003). Evaluation of anthropometric, physiological, and skill-related tests for talent identification in female field hockey. *Canadian Journal of Applied Physiology, 28*(3), 397–409.

Roetert, E. P., Brown, S. W., Piorkowski, P. A., & Woods, R. B. (1996). Fitness comparisons among three different levels of elite tennis players. *Journal of Strength and Conditioning Research, 10*(3), 139–143.

Roetert, E. P., Piorkowski, P. A., Woods, R. B., & Brown, S. W. (1995). Establishing percentiles for junior tennis players based on physical fitness testing results. *Clinics in Sports Medicine, 14*(1), 1–21.

Suni, J. A., Miilunpalo, S. I., Asikainen, T. M., et al. (1998). Safety and feasibility of a health-related fitness test battery for adults. *Physical Therapy, 78*(2), 134–148.

Tan, B., Aziz, A. R., Teh, K. C., & Lee, H. C. (2001). Grip strength measurement in competitive ten-pin bowlers. *Journal of Sports and Medicine in Physical Fitness, 41*(1), 68–72.

Xio, G., Lei, L., Dempsey, P. G., Lu, B., & Liang, Y. (2005). Isometric muscle strength and anthropometric characteristics of a Chinese sample. *International Journal of Industrial Ergonomics, 35,* 674–679.

■ 1-REPETITION MAXIMUM (1RM) BENCH PRESS TEST

Objective: Measure absolute or relative upper-body strength

Age Range: High school to adult

Equipment Needed:

1. Weight bench
2. Wide selection of barbell weight plates
3. Calibrated scale (only necessary to determine relative upper body strength)

Additional Personnel Needed: One to three test assistants (spotters)

Setup:

1. For all bench press testing, the test performer assumes the proper bench press position by lying supine with both feet flat on the floor and grasps the bar with a closed, pronated grip slightly wider than shoulder width apart. The test performer must utilize proper technique for all trials.
2. For all bench press testing, each test assistant assumes the proper bench press spotting position and utilizes proper spotting techniques (**Figure 6-3**). Based on the ability of the test performer and spotter(s), one, two, or three spotter(s) may be needed for each bench press attempt.

Administration and Directions:

1. The test administrator instructs the test performer to warm up by utilizing light resistance that *easily* allows the test performer to complete 5 to 10 repetitions.
2. The test performer is given a 1-minute rest.
3. The test administrator estimates a load that will allow the test performer to complete 3 to 5 bench press repetitions. This may be a 10- to 20-pound (4.5- to 9-kilogram) or 5% to 10% weight increase.

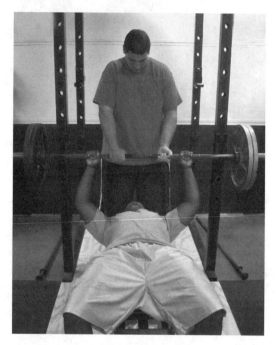

Figure 6-3   1-Repetition Maximum Bench Press Test Setup

4. The test performer is given a 2-minute rest.
5. The test administrator estimates a *conservative* load that will result in a near-maximal load allowing the test performer to complete 2 or 3 bench press repetitions. This may be a 10- to 20-pound (4.5- to 9-kilogram) or 5% to 10% weight increase.
6. The test performer is given a 2- to 4-minute rest.
7. The test administrator makes a load increase by 10 to 20 pounds (4.5 to 9 kilograms) or 5% to 10%.
8. The test performer attempts a 1RM bench press.

9. *If the test performer's attempt is successful,* a 2- to 4-minute rest is provided. The test administrator goes back to step 7 and asks the test performer to make another repetition attempt.

10. *If the test performer's attempt is unsuccessful,* a 2- to 4-minute rest is provided. The test administrator reduces the load by 5 to 10 pounds (2.2- to 4.5-kg) or 2.5% to 5% before the test performer makes another 1RM attempt (go back to step 8).

11. This process of adding and subtracting weight is continued until the test performer can complete one maximum bench press repetition (with proper technique). This should be accomplished in 3 to 5 test repetitions.

Scoring:

1. Absolute strength: The heaviest weight lifted utilizing proper technique is recorded as the final score.

2. Relative strength: The amount of weight lifted utilizing proper technique when divided by the test performer's body weight is recorded as the final score.

relative strength = weight lifted ÷ body weight

It is advisable to record the test performer's 1RM bench press score and body weight separately.

Checklist: The test performer must

1. Utilize proper bench press techniques during all trials
2. Utilize proper communication techniques with the spotter(s)
3. Rest between trials

References

American College of Sports Medicine. (2006). *ACSM's guidelines for exercise testing and prescription* (7th ed.). Philadelphia: Lippincott Williams & Wilkins.

Baechle, T. R., & Earle, R. W. (2008). *Essentials of strength training and conditioning* (3rd ed.). Champaign, IL: Human Kinetics.

Chapman, P. P., Whitehead, J. R., & Binkert, R. H. (1998). The 225-lb reps-to-fatigue test as a submaximal estimate of 1-RM bench press performance in college football players. *Journal of Strength and Conditioning Research, 12*(4), 258–261.

Gore, C. J. (2000). *Physiological tests for elite athletes.* Australian Sports Commission. Champaign, IL: Human Kinetics.

Heyward, V. H. (2006). *Advanced fitness assessment and exercise prescription* (5th ed.). Champaign, IL: Human Kinetics.

Johnson, B. L., & Nelson, J. K. (1986). *Practical measurements for evaluation in physical education* (4th ed.). New York: MacMillan.

Mayhew, J. L., Bemben, M. G., Rohrs, D. M., Ware, J., & Bemben, D. A. (1991). Seated shot put as a measure of upper body power in college males. *Journal of Human Movement Studies, 21*(3), 137–148.

Mayhew, J. L., Ware, J. S., Bemben, M. G., Wilt, B., et al. (1999). The NFL-225 test as a measure of bench press strength in college football players. *Journal of Strength and Conditioning Research, 13*(2), 130–134.

Mayhew, J. L., Ware, J. S., Cannon, K., Corbett, S., et al. (2002). Validation of the NFL-225 test for predict 1-RM bench press performance in college football players. *Journal of Sports and Medicine in Physical Fitness, 42*(3), 304–308.

Nesser, T. W., Huxel, K. C., Tincher, J. L., & Okada, T. (2008). The relationship between core stability and performance in division I football players. *Journal of Strength and Conditioning Research, 22*(6), 1750–1754.

Semenick, D. (1981). Conditioning program: Testing and evaluation. *National Strength and Conditioning Association Journal, 3*(2), 8–9.

Tritschler, K. (2000). *Barrow & McGee's Practical Measurement and Assessment* Philadelphia: Lippincott Williams & Wilkins.

■ 1-REPETITION MAXIMUM (1RM) SQUAT TEST

Objective: Measure absolute or relative lower-body strength

Age Range: High school to adult

Equipment Needed:

1. Squat rack
2. Wide selection of weight plates
3. Calibrated scale (necessary only to determine relative lower-body strength)

Additional Personnel Needed: Two or three test assistants (spotters)

Setup:

1. For all squat testing, the test performer assumes the proper squat position by grasping the bar with a closed, pronated grip and stepping under the bar. The feet should be positioned parallel to each other and shoulder width apart. The chest should be held up and out and the head tilted up slightly. The hips and knees should extend to lift the bar. Once the bar is lifted, the test performer takes one or two steps backward and positions the feet shoulder width apart with the toes slightly pointed outward (**Figure 6-4**).
2. For all squat testing, each test assistant assumes the proper squat spotting position(s) and utilizes proper spotting techniques. Based on the abilities of the test performer and spotters, two or three spotters may be needed for each squat attempt.

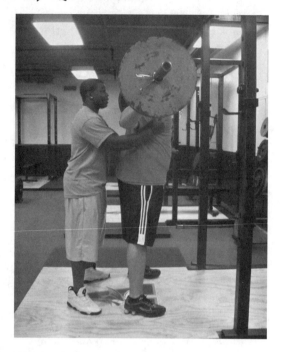

Figure 6-4   1-Repetition Maximum Squat Test Setup

Administration and Directions:

1. The test administrator instructs the test performer to warm up by utilizing light resistance that allows the test performer to *easily* complete 5 to 10 squat repetitions.
2. The test performer is given a one-minute rest.

3. The test administrator estimates a load that will allow the test performer to complete 3 to 5 squat repetitions. This may be a 30- to 40-pound (13.6- to 18.1-kilogram) or 10% to 20% weight increase.
4. The test performer is given a 2-minute rest.
5. The test administrator estimates a *conservative* load that will result in a near-maximal load allowing the test performer to complete 2 or 3 squat repetitions. This may be a 30- to 40-pound (13.6- to 18.1-kilogram) 10% to 20% weight increase.
6. The test performer is given a 2- to 4-minute rest.

7. The test administrator increases the load by 30 to 40 pounds (13.6 to 18.1 kilograms) or 10% to 20%.

8. The test performer attempts a 1RM squat.

9. *If the test performer's attempt is successful*, a 2- to 4-minute rest is provided. The test administrator goes back to step 7 and asks the test performer to make another repetition attempt.

10. *If the test performer's attempt is unsuccessful*, a 2- to 4-minute rest is provided. The test administrator reduces the load by 15 to 20 pounds (6.8 to 9 kg) or 5% to 10% before the test performer makes another 1RM attempt (go back to step 8).

11. This process of adding and subtracting weight is continued until the test performer can complete one maximum squat repetition (with proper technique). This should be accomplished in 3 to 5 test repetitions.

Scoring:

1. Absolute strength: The heaviest weight lifted utilizing proper technique is recorded as the final score.

2. Relative strength: The amount of weight lifted utilizing proper technique when divided by the test performer's body weight is recorded as the final score.

relative strength = weight lifted ÷ body weight

It is advisable to record the test performer's 1RM squat score and body weight separately.

Checklist: The test performer must

1. Utilize proper squat technique during all trials

2. Utilize the same squat positions for all trials (front vs. back squat and low vs. high bar position)

3. Utilize proper communication with the spotters

4. Rest between trials

References

American College of Sports Medicine. (2006). *ACSM's guidelines for exercise testing and prescription* (7th ed.). Philadelphia: Lippincott Williams & Wilkins.

Baechle, T. R., & Earle, R. W. (2008). *Essentials of strength training and conditioning* (3rd ed.). Champaign, IL: Human Kinetics.

Gore, C. J. (2000). *Physiological tests for elite athletes*. Australian Sports Commission. Champaign, IL: Human Kinetics.

Johnson, B. L., & Nelson, J. K. (1986). *Practical measurements for evaluation in physical education* (4th ed.). New York: MacMillan.

Murphy, A. J., & Wilson, G. J. (1997). The ability of tests of muscular function to reflect training-induced changes in performance. *Journal of Sports Sciences, 15*, 191–200.

Nesser, T. W., Huxel, K. C., Tincher, J. L., & Okada, T. (2008). The relationship between core stability and performance in division I football flayers. *Journal of Strength and Conditioning Research, 22*(6), 1750–1754.

Newton, R. U., Gerber, A., Nimphius, S., Shim, J. K., et al. (2006). Determination of functional strength imbalance of the lower extremities. Journal of Strength and Conditioning Research, 20(4), 971–977.

Semenick, D. (1981). Conditioning program: Testing and evaluation. National Strength and Conditioning Association Journal, 3(2), 8–9.

■ SIT-UPS FOR STRENGTH TEST

Objective: Measure the strength of the abdominal muscles during trunk flexion

Age Range: 12 to college age

Equipment Needed:

1. Exercise mat(s)
2. Plate weights or dumbbells
3. Ruler
4. Tape or chalk

Additional Personnel Needed: Two test assistants

Setup:

1. The test performer selects the amount of weight he or she wants to use during the sit-up. The weight chosen (especially for the first attempt) should be relatively light.
2. A straight line is created on one end of the exercise mat with tape or chalk.
3. The test performer assumes a supine position with the buttocks just above the line, with the knees slightly flexed and feet flat on the exercise mat.
4. A test assistant places a ruler behind the test performer's knees.

5. The test performer then flexes the knees until he or she can hold the ruler securely behind the knees with the legs.
6. The test performer then slowly extends the knees by sliding the feet forward until the ruler falls.
7. Once the ruler falls, the test administrator places a mark at the heels of the test performer with a strip of tape or chalk. This is the starting position for this test performer.
8. A test assistant places the chosen weight behind the test performer's head and neck. It should be firmly grasped by the test performer. A second test assistant stabilizes the test performer's feet with the test performer in the determined starting position (**Figure 6-5**).

Administration and Directions:

1. On the test administrator's "go" command, the test performer attempts to execute a single sit-up from the determined starting position. The sit-up is considered complete when the test performer's elbows touch the thighs (**Figure 6-6**).

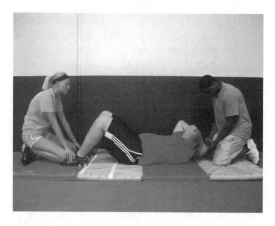

Figure 6-5 Sit-Ups for Strength Test Setup

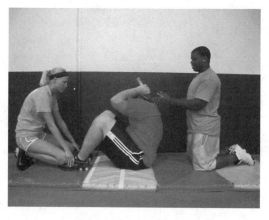

Figure 6-6 Sit-Ups for Strength Test Administration

2. The test administrator (or test assistant) should remove the weight from behind the test performer's head once the sit-up attempt is completed (successfully or unsuccessfully).
3. The weight may be adjusted (heavier or lighter) and the same protocol used on the subsequent trial.
4. A maximum of two trials are performed.

Scoring: The greatest amount of weight successfully lifted is recorded as the final score.

Checklist: The test performer must

1. Maintain the proper sit-up position during each attempt
2. Not choose a weight that is obviously too heavy (especially on the first trial)
3. Not attempt to return to the exercise mat after the sit-up attempt (successful or unsuccessful) until the test administrator (or a designated test assistant) safely removes the weight from the back of the test performer's head and neck
4. If the weight cannot be removed safely, the test performer must release his or grip and allow the weight to drop to the exercise mat before returning to the exercise mat

References

Johnson, B. L., & Nelson, J. K. (1986). *Practical measurements for evaluation in physical education* (4th ed.). New York: MacMillan.

Miller, D. K. (2006). *Measurement by the physical educator: Why and how* (5th ed.). New York: McGraw-Hill.

■ ABDOMINAL STAGE TEST

Objective: Measure abdominal strength in stages

Age Range: High school to college age

Equipment Needed:

1. Flat floor or exercise mat
2. 2.5-kilogram (5.5-pound) plate weight
3. 5-kilogram (11-pound) plate weight

Additional Personnel Needed: Test assistant

Setup:

1. The test performer removes his or her shoes and lays supine on the floor with the knees bent to 90°. The feet should not be held. This is the starting position for each stage (**Figure 6-7**).

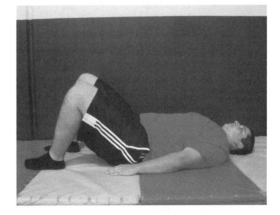

Figure 6-7 Abdominal Stage Test Setup

2. The test administrator explains to the test performer that each stage must be completed before he or she is allowed to move onto the subsequent stage, and the test performer cannot deviate from the proper sit-up protocol (described below). Each stage must be completed in a smooth, controlled manner.

Administration and Directions:

1. Stage 1 (palms over knees): The test performer extends the elbows and places the palms flat on the thighs. The test performer then moves forward until the fingers touch the patella (**Figure 6-8**).

2. Stage 2 (elbows over knees): The test performer extends the elbows and places the palms flat on the thighs. The test performer then moves forward until the elbows touch the patella (**Figure 6-9**).

3. Stage 3 (forearms to thighs): The test performer crosses the arms on the abdomen. The test performer then moves forward until the forearms touch the thigh (**Figure 6-10**).

4. Stage 4 (elbows to thighs): The test performer crosses his or her arms with the right hand touching the left shoulder and vice versa. The test performer then moves forward until the elbows touch the thighs (**Figure 6-11**).

5. Stage 5 (chest to thighs): The test performer bends the arms behind the head with the right hand touching the back of the left shoulder and vice versa. The test performer then moves forward until the chest touches the thighs (**Figure 6-12**).

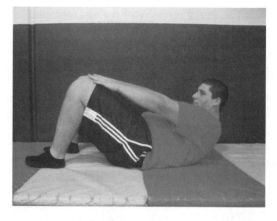

Figure 6-8   Abdominal Stage Test: Stage 1

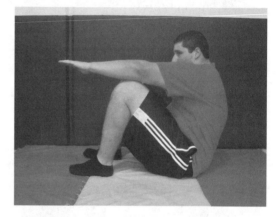

Figure 6-9   Abdominal Stage Test: Stage 2

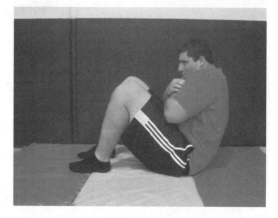

Figure 6-10   Abdominal Stage Test: Stage 3

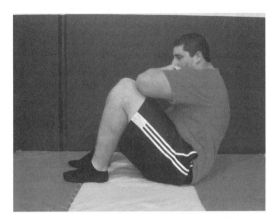

Figure 6-11 Abdominal Stage Test: Stage 4

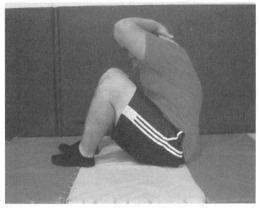

Figure 6-12 Abdominal Stage Test: Stage 5

6. Stage 6 (chest to thighs with 2.5-kilogram/5.5-pound weight): The test performer places the hands in the same position as in stage 5. The test assistant places a 2.5-kilogram (5.5-pound) weight between the test performer's hands. The test performer grasps and holds the weight. The test performer then moves forward until the chest touches the thighs (**Figure 6-13**). The test assistant may

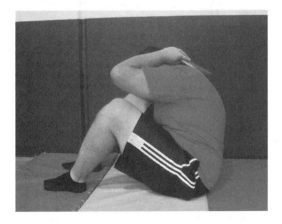

Figure 6-13 Abdominal Stage Test: Stages 6 and 7

need to secure the weight once the test performer completes or fails the trial.

7. Stage 7 (chest to thighs with 5-kilogram/11-pound weight): The same protocol used in stage 6 is followed, but the test performer uses a 5-kilogram (11-pound) weight. (Refer to Figure 6-13.)

8. The test performer may make three attempts to complete each stage before the test is discontinued.

9. One complete abdominal stage test is performed.

Scoring:

1. An attempt does not count if the test performer does any of the following during a trial.
   a. Lifts either foot from the ground
   b. Throws or jerks the head forward violently
   c. Moves the arms from the designated position
   d. Lifts the hips off the floor
   e. Fails to maintain the knees at a 90° angle
   f. Is unable to complete the sit-up successfully

2. Each stage is recorded as pass or fail.

3. The highest stage the test performer completes is recorded as the final score.

Checklist: The test performer must

1. Be in the correct starting position for each attempt
2. Not have the feet held
3. Complete each stage successfully before moving onto the subsequent stage

Reference

Gore, C. J. (2000). *Physiological tests for elite athletes.* Australian Sports Commission. Champaign, IL: Human Kinetics.

■ PULL-UPS FOR STRENGTH TEST

Objective: Measure upper-body strength

Age Range: 12 to college age

Equipment Needed:

1. Horizontal bar
2. Chair
3. Calibrated scale
4. Variety of plate weights and ropes or straps to secure the weights to the waist of the test performer *or*
5. Weight vest with a variety of weights

Additional Personnel Needed: Test assistant

Setup:

1. The test performer is weighed on the calibrated scale.
2. The horizontal bar is adjusted to a height where the test performer's feet will be off the floor.
3. A weight is selected that the test performer believes he or she can lift. The weight is secured to the test performer's waist or the weight vest.
4. The test performer stands on the chair (secured by the test assistant) and grasps the horizontal bar with the palms forward (overhand grip) (**Figure 6-14**).

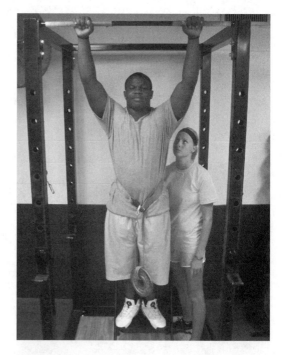

Figure 6-14 Pull-Ups for Strength Test Setup

5. When the test performer gives the ready signal, the test assistant removes the chair and the test performer lowers the body to the starting position with the elbows straight (**Figure 6-15**).

Administration and Directions:

1. On the test administrator's "go" command, the test performer attempts to pull the chin over the horizontal bar (**Figure 6-16**).
2. Once the attempt is deemed successful or unsuccessful, the test assistant places the chair back under the test performer so he or she can safely come down from the horizontal bar.

3. The weight is adjusted (heavier or lighter) if necessary and the same protocol used on the subsequent trial.
4. Two trials are permitted.

Scoring:

1. The greatest amount of weight successfully lifted is recorded.
2. The final score is the amount of weight successfully lifted divided by the test performer's body weight.

relative strength = weight lifted ÷ body weight

3. If a test performer cannot lift more than his or her body weight, a score of 0 is given.

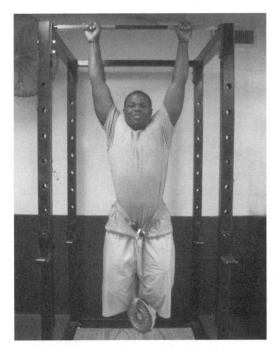

Figure 6-15   Pull-Ups for Strength Test Starting Position

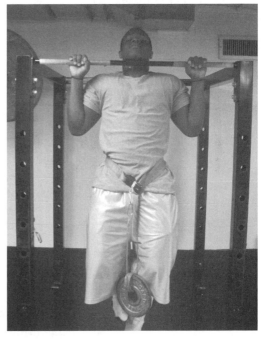

Figure 6-16   Pull-Ups for Strength Test Administration

Checklist: The test performer must

1. Not swing the body (or the weight) during the test
2. Securely place both feet on the chair before releasing his or her grip on the horizontal bar

References

Johnson, B. L., & Nelson, J. K. (1986). *Practical measurements for evaluation in physical education* (4th ed.). New York: MacMillan.

Miller, D. K. (2006). *Measurement by the physical educator: Why and how* (5th ed.). New York: McGraw-Hill.

■ DIPS FOR STRENGTH TEST

Objective: Measure upper-body strength

Age Range: 12 to college age

Equipment Needed:

1. Horizontal bar
2. Chair
3. Calibrated scale
4. Variety of plate weights and ropes or straps to secure the weights to the waist of the test performer *or*
5. Weight vest with a variety of weights

Additional Personnel Needed: Test assistant

Setup:

1. The test performer is weighed on the calibrated scale.
2. The parallel bars are adjusted to a height where the test performer's feet will be off the ground while in the bent-arm position.
3. The test performer selects a weight. The weight is secured to the test performer's waist or the weight vest.
4. The test performer stands on the chair (secured by the test assistant) and grasps the parallel bars securely (**Figure 6-17**).
5. When the test performer gives the ready signal, the test assistant removes the chair and the test performer remains in the straight-arm starting position (**Figure 6-18**).

Administration and Directions:

1. On the test administrator's "go" command, the test performer lowers his or her body

until the elbows form a 90° angle; this is the bent-arm position (**Figure 6-19**).

2. Once the bent-arm position is achieved, the test performer extends the elbows and returns to a straight-arm position.
3. Once the attempt is deemed successful or unsuccessful, the test assistant places the chair back under the test performer so

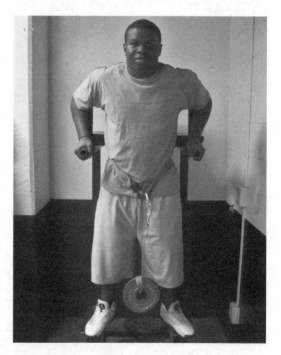

Figure 6-17 Dips for Strength Test Setup

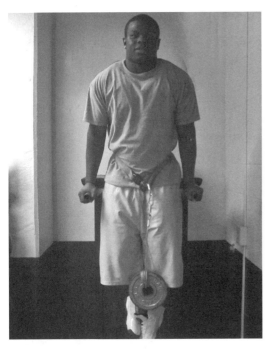

Figure 6-18 Dips for Strength Test Starting Position

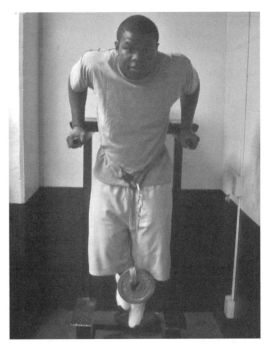

Figure 6-19 Dips for Strength Test Administration

that he or she can safely come down from the parallel bars.

4. The weight may be adjusted (heavier or lighter) and the same protocol used on a subsequent trial.
5. Two trials are permitted.

Scoring:

1. The greatest amount of weight successfully lifted is recorded.
2. The final score is the amount of weight successfully lifted divided by the test performer's body weight.

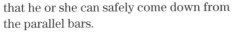

relative strength = weight lifted ÷ body weight

3. If the test performer cannot lift more than his or her body weight, a score of 0 is given.

Checklist: The test performer must

1. Not swing the body (or the weight) during the test
2. Securely place both feet on the chair before releasing his or her grip on the parallel bars

References

Johnson, B. L., & Nelson, J. K. (1986). *Practical measurements for evaluation in physical education* (4th ed.). New York: MacMillan.

Miller, D. K. (2006). *Measurement by the physical educator: Why and how* (5th ed.). New York: McGraw-Hill.

CHAPTER 7

Power Testing

Power testing, also termed anaerobic power, is the ability of the body or muscular group to exert high force at a fast rate. Muscular power is also thought of as explosiveness. Muscular power tests occur over a short time span and at maximum movement speed, requiring about 1 second to complete.

Proper technique and experience are essential to performing muscular power tests correctly and without injury. The test administrator should ensure that the test performer demonstrates proper technique before any power test is conducted. Having the test performer warm up with light (or no) weight allows the test administrator to ensure the performer has proper technique while providing the test performer practice for the test. The test administrator should provide the test performer with adequate rest between trials, allowing the test performer's muscles to regenerate energy stores. Muscular power tests are not considered a component of good general health and fitness; however, muscular power tests are important considerations for the evaluation of athletic talent and abilities. Muscular power testing is normally performed solely on athletes. Muscular power tests should be performed early in a test battery before excessive fatigue is experienced.

■ STANDING BROAD JUMP TEST

Also Known as: Standing Long Jump Test

Objective: Measure lower-body horizontal power

Age Range: 6 to college age

Equipment Needed:

1. Athletic tape (or a solid line)
2. Tape measure
3. Measuring stick
4. Long-jump pit and rake (preferable) *or*
5. Open gym or outdoor surface

Additional Personnel Needed: Test assistant

Setup:

1. The test administrator places a strip of tape where the test performer will jump from, or makes use of an existing solid line.
2. The test administrator unrolls the tape measure and places it along the side where the test performer will land. The tape measure may be secured to the floor with tape.
3. The test performer stands behind the starting line, with the feet parallel and shoulder width apart.

Administration and Directions:

1. On the test administrator's "go" command, the test performer bends the knees, swings the arms, and jumps forward as far as possible (**Figure 7-1**).
2. The test performer should remain stationary after landing so the attempt can be measured. If a long-jump pit is used, the test performer does not need to remain stationary after landing. The long-jump pit should be raked between attempts.
3. Up to three trials are performed.

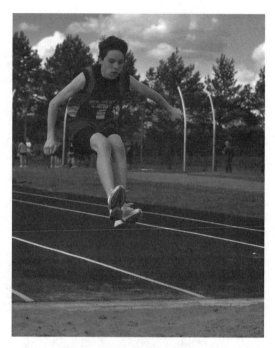

Figure 7-1   Standing Broad Jump Test Administration

Scoring:

1. Once the test performer lands, the test administrator places the measuring stick perpendicular to the test performer's *nearest heel* to the starting line. The measurement is recorded from that mark to the front of the starting line.
2. If the test performer falls backward upon landing, the measurement is taken from the body part closest to the starting line.
3. Each attempt is recorded.
4. The longest jump is recorded as the final score.

Checklist: The test performer must

1. Begin the jump with both feet completely behind the starting line
2. Not move after landing from the jump unless he or she jumps into a long-jump pit

References

American Association for Health, Physical Education, Recreation, and Dance (AAHPERD). (1976). *AAHPER youth fitness test manual.* Washington, DC: AAHPERD.

Baechle, T. R., & Earle, R. W. (2008). *Essentials of strength training and conditioning* (3rd ed.). Champaign, IL: Human Kinetics.

Brodie, D. A. (1996). *A reference manual for human performance measurement in the field of physical education and sports sciences.* Lewiston, NY: Edwin Mellen Press.

Coaches roundtable: Testing for football. (1983). *National Strength and Conditioning Association Journal, 5*(5), 12–19.

Farlinger, C. M., Kruisselbrink, L. D., & Fowles, J. R. (2007). Relationships to skating performance in competitive hockey players. *Journal of Strength and Conditioning Research, 21*(3), 915–922.

Glencross, D. J. (1966). The nature of the vertical jump test and the standing broad jump. *Research Quarterly, 37*(3), 353–359.

Gore, C. J. (2000). *Physiological tests for elite athletes.* Australian Sports Commission. Champaign, IL: Human Kinetics.

Huang, Y. C., & Malina, R. M. (2007). BMI and health-related physical fitness in Taiwanese youth 9–19 years. *Medicine and Science in Sports and Exercise, 39*(4), 701–708.

Inside the Combine. (2008, February 20). *Chicago Tribune,* 5–7.

Johnson, B. L., & Nelson, J. K. (1986). *Practical measurements for evaluation in physical education* (4th ed.). New York: MacMillan.

Keough, J. W. L., Weber, C. L., & Dalton, C. T. (2003). Evaluation of anthropometric, physiological, and skill-related tests for talent identification in female field hockey. *Canadian Journal of Applied Physiology, 28*(3), 397–409.

Kuzmits, F. E., & Adams, A. J. (2008). The NFL combine: Does it predict performance in the National Football League? *Journal of Strength and Conditioning Research, 22*(6), 1721–1727.

Mayhew, J. L., Bemben, M. G., Rohrs, D. M., & Bemben, D. A. (1994). Specificity among anaerobic power tests in college female athletes. *Journal of Strength and Conditioning Research, 8*(1), 43–47.

Markovic, G., Dizdar, D., Jukic, I., & Cardinale, M. (2004). Reliability and factorial validity of squat and countermovement jump tests. *Journal of Strength and Conditioning Research, 18*(3), 551–555.

McGee, K. J., & Burkett, L. N. (2003). The National Football League combine: A reliable predictor of draft status. *Journal of Strength and Conditioning Research, 17*(1), 6–11.

McSwegin, P., Pemberton, C., Petray, C., & Going, S. (1989). *Physical best: The AAHPERD guide to physical fitness education and assessment.* Reston, VA: AAHPERD.

Miller, D. K. (2006). *Measurement by the physical educator: Why and how* (5th ed.). New York: McGraw-Hill.

Safrit, M. J. (1995). *Complete guide to youth fitness testing.* Champaign, IL: Human Kinetics.

Sierer, S. P., Battaglini, C. L., Mihalik, J. P., Shields, E. W., & Tomasini, N. T. (2008). The National Football League Combine: Performance differences between drafted and nondrafted players entering the 2004 and 2005 drafts. *Journal of Strength and Conditioning Research, 22*(1), 6–12.

Wiklander, J., & Lysholm, J. (1987). Simple tests for surveying muscle strength and muscle stiffness in sportsmen. *International Journal of Sports Medicine, 8*(1), 50–54.

■ SARGENT'S TEST

Also Known as: Vertical Jump Test: Wall Method

Objective: Measure lower-body vertical power

Age Range: 9 to adult

Equipment Needed:

1. Measuring tape or measuring stick
2. Chalk (either a stick of chalk or powdered chalk)
3. High wall
4. White athletic tape

Additional Personnel Needed: None

Setup:

1. The measuring tape or measuring stick is secured to the wall vertically from a fixed point (i.e., 48 inches above the floor), or a vertically taped and marked line may be secured to the wall.
2. The test performer stands approximately 6 inches (15 centimeters) from the wall with the preferred arm (the arm the performer writes with) toward the wall and the feet flat on the floor.
3. The test performer is given chalk.
4. The test performer reaches as high as possible with the feet flat on the floor and makes a horizontal mark on the wall with the chalk (**Figure 7-2**). This is the test performer's standing vertical reach (SVR).

Administration and Directions:

1. On the test administrator's "go" command, the test performer lowers the preferred arm, and without a preparatory (stutter) step, performs a countermovement jump (**Figure 7-3**).
2. The test performer should swing the preferred arm upward while keeping the non-preferred arm down.
3. The test performer makes another chalk mark (jump height) on the wall with the

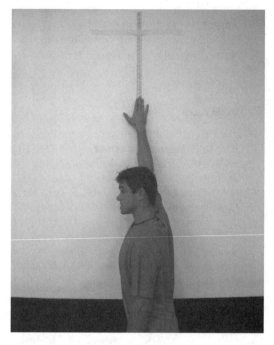

Figure 7-2 Sargent's Test Setup

preferred hand when the highest vertical point is reached.

4. This same protocol can be utilized to measure a test performer's one-leg vertical jump height.
5. Three trials are performed.

Scoring: The test administrator measures the distance between the SVR and the highest chalk mark. The SVR height is subtracted from the vertical jump (VJ) height and recorded as the final score.

VJ – SVR

Checklist: The test performer must

1. Practice the movement before the trial begins

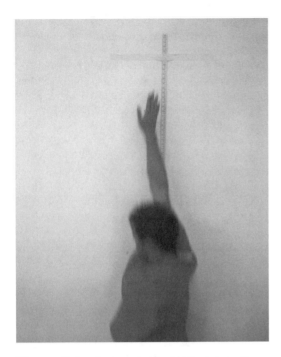

Figure 7-3 Sargent's Test Administration

2. Utilize the same jumping motion on each trial and subsequent tests
3. Not take a stutter-step before jumping

References

Baechle, T. R., & Earle, R. W. (2008). *Essentials of strength training and conditioning* (3rd ed.). Champaign, IL: Human Kinetics.

Bandy, W. D., Rusche, K. R., & Tekulve, F. Y. (1994). Reliability and limb symmetry for five unilateral functional tests of the lower extremities. *Isokinetics and Exercise Science, 4*(3), 108–111.

Barnekow-Bergkvist, M., Hedberg, G., Janlert, U., & Jansson, E. (1996). Development of muscular endurance and strength from adolescence to adulthood and level of physical capacity in men and women at the age of 34 years. *Scandinavian Journal of Medicine, Science, and Sports, 6*, 145–155.

Brodie, D. A. (1996). *A reference manual for human performance measurement in the field of physical education and sports sciences.* Lewiston, NY: Edwin Mellen Press.

Coaches roundtable: Testing for football. (1983). *National Strength and Conditioning Association Journal, 5*(5), 12–19.

Gabbett, T., & Georgieff, B. (2007). Physiological and anthropometric characteristics of Australian junior national, state, and novice volleyball players. *Journal of Strength and Conditioning Research, 21*(3), 902–908.

Glencross, D. J. (1966). The nature of the vertical jump test and the standing broad jump. *Research Quarterly, 37*(3), 353–359.

Gore, C. J. (2000). *Physiological tests for elite athletes.* Australian Sports Commission. Champaign, IL: Human Kinetics.

Johnson, B. L., & Nelson, J. K. (1986). *Practical measurements for evaluation in physical education* (4th ed.). New York: MacMillan.

Keough, J. W. L., Weber, C. L., & Dalton, C. T. (2003). Evaluation of anthropometric, physiological, and skill-related tests for talent identification in female field hockey. *Canadian Journal of Applied Physiology, 28*(3), 397–409.

Roetert, E. P., Brown, S. W., Piorkowski, P. A., & Woods, R. B. (1996). Fitness comparisons among three different levels of elite tennis players. *Journal of Strength and Conditioning Research, 10*(3), 139–143.

Rosch, D., Hodgson, R., Peterson, L., Graf-Baumann, T., Junge, A., Chomiak, J., & Dvorak, J. (2000). Assessment and evaluation of football performance. *American Journal of Sports Medicine, 28*(5), S29–S40.

Sargent, D. A. (1921). The physical test of a man. *American Physical Education Review, 26*(4), 188–194.

Semenick, D. (1984). Anaerobic testing: Practical applications. *National Strength and Conditioning Association Journal, 6*(5), 45, 70–73.

Semenick, D. (1981). Conditioning program: Testing and evaluation. *National Strength and Conditioning Association Journal, 3*(2), 8–9.

Semenick, D. (1990). Tests and measurements: The vertical jump. *National Strength and Conditioning Association Journal, 12*(3), 68–69.

Semenick, D., Connors, J., Carter, M., Harman, E., et al. (1992). Test and measurement: Rationale, protocols, testing/reporting forms and instructions for wrestling. *National Strength and Conditioning Association Journal, 14* (3), 54–59.

Tritschler, K. (2000). *Barrow & McGee's practical measurement and assessment* (5th ed.). Philadelphia: Lippincott Williams & Wilkins.

■ VANE-SLAT APPARATUS METHOD

Also Known as: Vertical Jump Test

Objective: Measure lower-body vertical power

Age Range: 9 to adult

Equipment Needed:

1. Commercially available vane-slat apparatus (i.e., Vertec®)
2. Measuring stick

Additional Personnel Needed: None

Setup:

1. The test performer's standing vertical reach (SVR) is determined by having him or her stand with feet flat on the ground and reach with the preferred hand (the hand the performer writes with) while the test administrator adjusts the height of the lowest vane to be at the same height as the test performer's standing reach (**Figure 7-4**).
2. The test administrator records the height.
3. The test administrator then raises the vane stack so the test performer will not jump higher than the vane stack.

Administration and Directions:

1. On the test administrator's "go" command, the test performer lowers the preferred arm, and without a preparatory (stutter) step, performs a countermovement jump (**Figure 7-5**).

2. The test performer should swing the preferred arm upward while keeping the non-preferred arm down.

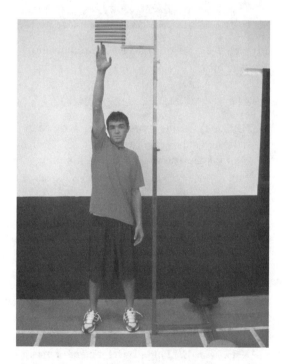

Figure 7-4   Vane-Slat Apparatus Method Setup

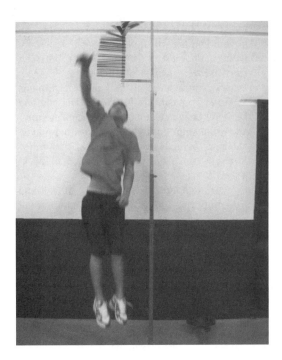

Figure 7-5 Vane-Slat Apparatus Method Administration

3. The test performer displaces as many vanes as possible when the highest vertical point is reached.
4. The test administrator may need to adjust the height of the vane stack based on the vertical jumping ability of the test performer.
5. After each trial, the test administrator records the jump height and resets the vanes with the measuring stick.
6. The height of the vertical jump is determined by adding the number on the side of the vane-slat apparatus with the number of vanes displaced to the nearest 0.5 inches (1.24 centimeters). Each vane represents 0.5 inches (1.24 centimeters) of vertical height.
7. Three trials are preformed.

Scoring: The SVR is subtracted from the vertical jump (VJ) and recorded as the final score.

$$VJ - SVR$$

Checklist: The test performer must

1. Practice the movement before the trial begins
2. Utilize the same jumping motion on each trial and subsequent tests
3. Not take a stutter-step before jumping

References

Baechle, T. R., & Earle, R. W. (2008). *Essentials of strength training and conditioning* (3rd ed.). Champaign, IL: Human Kinetics.

Burkett, L. N., Phillips, W. T., & Ziuraitis, J. (2005). The best warm-up for the vertical jump in college-age athletic men. *Journal of Strength and Conditioning Research, 19*(3), 673–676.

Coaches roundtable: Testing for football. (1983). *National Strength and Conditioning Association Journal, 5*(5), 12–19.

Davis, D. S., Barnette, B. J., Kiger, J. T., Mirasola, J. J., & Young, S. M. (2004). Physical characteristics that predict functional performance in Division I college football players. *Journal of Strength and Conditioning Research, 18*(1), 115–120.

Farlinger, C. M., Kruisselbrink, L. D., & Fowles, J. R. (2007). Relationships to skating performance in competitive hockey players. *Journal of Strength and Conditioning Research, 21*(3), 915–922.

Gore, C. J. (2000). *Physiological tests for elite athletes.* Australian Sports Commission. Champaign, IL: Human Kinetics.

Kuzmits, F. E., & Adams, A. J. (2008). The NFL Combine: Does it predict performance in the National Football League? *Journal of Strength and Conditioning Research, 22*(6), 1721–1727.

McGee, K. J., & Burkett, L. N. (2003). The National Football League Combine: A reliable predictor of draft status. *Journal of Strength and Conditioning Research, 17*(1), 6–11.

Nesser, T. W., Huxel, K. C., Tincher, J. L., & Okada, T. (2008). The relationship between core stability and performance in Division I football players. *Journal of Strength and Conditioning Research, 22*(6), 1750–1754.

Patterson, D. D., & Peterson, D. F. (2004). Vertical jump and leg power norms for young adults. *Measurement in Physical Education and Exercise Science, 8*(1), 33–41.

Pauole, K., Madole, K., Garhammer, J., Lacourse, M., & Rozenek, R. (2000). Reliability and validity of the T-test as a measure of agility, leg power, and leg speed in college-aged men and women. *Journal of Strength and Conditioning Research, 14*(4), 443–450.

Sierer, S. P., Battaglini, C. L., Mihalik, J. P., Shields, E. W., & Tomasini, N. T. (2008). The National Football League Combine: Performance differences between drafted and nondrafted players entering the 2004 and 2005 drafts. *Journal of Strength and Conditioning Research, 22*(1), 6–12.

White, A. T., & Johnson, S. C. (1991). Physiological comparison of international, national and regional alpine skiers. *International Journal of Sports Medicine, 12*(4), 374–378.

■ 1-LEG HOP TEST

Also Known as: 1-Leg Hop for Distance (OLHD) Test

Objective: Measure lower-body horizontal power; this test can be used to examine ACL injuries and rehabilitation progress

Age Range: Child to adult

Equipment Needed:

1. Open grass field or gymnasium floor
2. Tape measure
3. Cone, tape, permanent line, or a similar marker to designate the starting point

Additional Personnel Needed: Test assistant

Setup:

1. The test performer stands behind the starting line and balances on one leg with the hands behind the back.
2. The test performer may practice the protocol (described as follows).

Administration and Directions:

1. On the test administrator's "go" command, the test performer, without taking a step backward, jumps forward as far as possible (**Figure 7-6**).
2. The test performer must land on the same foot he or she jumped from and is not required to maintain balance on the landing foot when landing.
3. However, if the test performer touches the ground with any other part of the body before the foot he or she jumped from, the trial is considered invalid and must be repeated.
4. Three trials are performed on each leg.

Scoring:

1. Each trial is measured from the starting line to the *heel* of the test performer's final landing position.

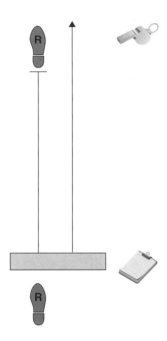

Figure 7-6 1-Leg Hop Test Administration

2. The final score can be recorded as the longest distance jumped on each foot or the average of the three trials on each foot.

Checklist: The test performer must

1. Not currently have a lower-body injury
2. Wear proper footwear for the surface the test is performed on
3. Have adequate balance before performing this test
4. Begin and end the test balancing on the same leg
5. Jump directly forward
6. Keep the hands behind the back during the test

References

Bandy, W. D., Rusche, K. R., & Tekulve, F. Y. (1994). Reliability and limb symmetry for five unilateral functional tests of the lower extrem-ities. *Isokinetics and Exercise Science, 4*(3), 108–111.

Bolgla, L. A., & Keskula, D. R. (1997). Reliability of lower extremity functional performance tests. *Journal of Orthopaedic and Sports Physical Therapy, 26*(3), 138–142.

Booher, L. D., Hench, K. M., Worrell, T. W., & Stikeleather, J. (1993). Reliability of three single-leg hop tests. *Journal of Sport Rehabilitation, 2*, 165–170.

Daniel, D. M., Stone, M. L., Riehl, B., & Moore, M. R. (1988). A measurement of lower limb function: The one leg hop for distance. *American Journal of Knee Surgery, 1*(4), 212–214.

Gustavsson, A., Neeter, C., Thomee, P., et al. (2006). A test battery for evaluating hop performance in patients with an ACL injury and patients who have undergone ACL reconstruction. *Knee Surgery, Sports Traumatology, Arthroscopy, 14*, 778–788.

Kramer, J. F., Nusca, D., Fowler, P., & Webster-Bogaert, S. (1992). Test-retest reliability of the one-leg hop test following ACL reconstruction. *Clinical Journal of Sports Medicine, 2*, 240–243.

Noyes, F. R., Barber, S. D., & Mangine, R. E. (1991). Abnormal lower limb symmetry determined by function hop tests after anterior cruciate ligament rupture. *American Journal of Sports Medicine, 19*(5), 513–518.

Nyberg, B., Granhed, H., Peterson, K., Piros, C., & Svantesson, U. (2006). Muscle strength and jumping distance during 10 years post ACL reconstruction. *Isokinetics and Exercise Science, 14*, 363–370.

O'Donnell, S., Thomas, S. G., & Marks, P. (2006). Improving the sensitivity of the hop index in patients with an ACL deficient knee by transforming the hop distance scores. *BMC Musculoskeletal Disorders (online), 7*, 9.

Ostenberg, A., Roos, E., Ekdahl, C., & Roos, H. (1998). Isokinetic knee extensor strength and functional performance in healthy female soccer players. *Scandinavian Journal of Medicine and Science in Sports, 8*, 257–264.

Petsching, R., Baron, R., & Albretcht, M. (1998). The relationship between isokinetic quadriceps strength test and hop tests for distance and one-legged vertical jump test following anterior cruciate ligament reconstruction. *Journal of Orthopaedic and Sports Physical Therapy*, *28*(1), 23–31.

Reid, A., Birmingham, T. B., Stratford, P. W., & Alcock, G. K. (2007). Hop testing provides a reliable and valid outcome measure during a rehabilitation after anterior cruciate ligament reconstruction. *Physical Therapy*, *87*(3), 337–349.

Ross, M. D., Langford, B., & Whelan, P. J. (2002). Test-retest reliability of four single-leg horizontal hop tests. *Journal of Strength and Conditioning Research*, *16*(4), 617–622.

Wilk, K. E., Romaniello, W. T., Soscia, S. M., Arrigo, C. A., & Andrews, J. A. (1994). The relationship between subjective knee scores, isokinetic testing, and functional testing in the ACL-reconstructed knee. *Journal of Orthopaedic and Sports Physical Therapy*, *20*(2), 60–73.

■ 3-HOP TEST

Also Known as: Triple-Hop (Jump) Test

Objective: Measure single-leg horizontal power

Age Range: High school to college age

Equipment Needed:

1. Open grass field or gymnasium floor
2. Tape measure
3. Cone, tape, permanent line, or a similar marker to designate the starting point

Additional Personnel Needed: Test assistant

Setup:

1. The test performer stands behind the starting line and balances on one leg.
2. The test performer may practice the protocol (described below).

Administration and Directions:

1. On the test administrator's "go" command, the test performer, without taking a step backward, jumps forward successively three times, landing on and jumping from the same leg (**Figure 7-7**).

2. The test performer should take three maximal hops forward.
3. If the test performer falls at any time during the trial or touches the ground with the non-balance leg, the trial is considered invalid and must be repeated.
4. Three trials are performed on each leg.

Scoring:

1. Each trial is measured from the starting line to the *heel* of the test performer's final landing position.
2. The average distance of the three trials is recorded as the final score.

Checklist: The test performer must

1. Not currently have a lower-body injury
2. Wear proper footwear for the surface the test is performed on
3. Have adequate balance before performing this test
4. Begin and end the test balancing on the same leg
5. Jump directly forward on each attempt

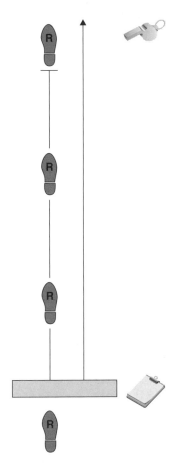

Figure 7-7 3-Hop Test Administration

References

Bandy, W. D., Rusche, K. R., & Tekulve, F. Y. (1994). Reliability and limb symmetry for five unilateral functional tests of the lower extremities. *Isokinetics and Exercise Science, 4*(3), 108–111.

Bolgla, L. A., & Keskula, D. R. (1997). Reliability of lower extremity functional performance tests. *Journal of Orthopaedic and Sports Physical Therapy, 26*(3), 138–142.

Farlinger, C. M., Kruisselbrink, L. D., & Fowles, J. R. (2007). Relationships to skating performance in competitive hockey players. *Journal of Strength and Conditioning Research, 21*(3), 915–922.

Hamilton, R. T., Schultz, S. J., Schmitz, R. J., & Perrin, D. H. (2008). Triple-hop distance as a valid predictor of lower limb strength and power. *Journal of Athletic Training, 43*(2), 144–151.

Noyes, F. R., Barber, S. D., & Mangine, R. E. (1991). Abnormal lower limb symmetry determined by function hop tests after anterior cruciate ligament rupture. *American Journal of Sports Medicine, 19*(5), 513–518.

Ostenberg, A., Roos, E., Ekdahl, C., & Roos, H. (1998). Isokinetic knee extensor strength and functional performance in healthy female soccer players. *Scandinavian Journal of Medicine and Science in Sports, 8*, 257–264.

Petsching, R., Baron, R., & Albretcht, M. (1998). The relationship between isokinetic quadriceps strength test and hop tests for distance and one-legged vertical jump test following anterior cruciate ligament reconstruction. *Journal of Orthopaedic and Sports Physical Therapy, 28*(1), 23–31.

Reid, A., Birmingham, T. B., Stratford, P. W., & Alcock, G. K. (2007). Hop testing provides a reliable and valid outcome measure during a rehabilitation after anterior cruciate ligament reconstruction. *Physical Therapy, 87*(3), 337–349.

Rosch, D., Hodgson, R., Peterson, L., Graf-Baumann, T., Junge, A., Chomiak, J., & Dvorak, J. (2000). Assessment and evaluation of football performance. *American Journal of Sports Medicine, 28*(5), S29–S40.

Ross, M. D., Langford, B., & Whelan, P. J. (2002). Test-retest reliability of four single-leg horizontal hop tests. *Journal of Strength and Conditioning Research, 16*(4), 617–622.

■ 5-JUMP TEST

Also Known as: 5-Hop Test

Objective: Measure lower-body power

Age Range: High school to college age

Equipment Needed:

1. Open grass field or gymnasium floor
2. Tape measure
3. Cone, tape, line, or a similar marker to designate the starting point

Additional Personnel Needed: Test assistant

Setup:

1. The test performer stands behind the starting line with the feet together.
2. The test performer may practice the protocol (described below).

Administration and Directions:

1. On the test administrator's "go" command, the test performer, without taking a step backward, jumps forward and lands on the foot of his or her choice (**Figure 7-8**).
2. The test performer then immediately jumps forward, landing on the *opposite* foot.
3. The process of jumping to opposing feet continues until the test performer lands on the left and right feet two times each, for a total of four jumps.
4. On the test performer's final jump, he or she lands with the feet together.
5. If the test performer falls at any time during the trial, the trial is considered invalid and repeated.
6. One trial is performed.

Scoring:

1. The trial is measured from the starting line to the *heel* of the test performer's final landing position.
2. The total distance traversed is recorded as the final score.

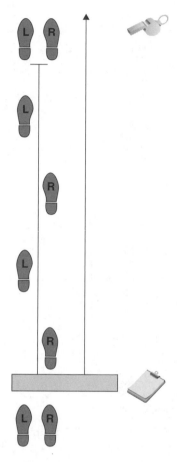

Figure 7-8 5-Jump Test Administration

Checklist: The test performer must

1. Not currently have a lower-body injury
2. Wear proper footwear for the surface the test is performed on
3. Begin and end the test with the feet joined together
4. Jump directly forward on each attempt

References

Chamari, K., Chaouachi, A., Hambli, M., Kaouech, F., Wisloff, U., & Castagna, C. (2008). The five-jump test for distance as a field test to assess lower limb explosive power in soccer players. *Journal of Strength and Conditioning Research, 22*(3), 944–950.

Chuman, K., Hoshikawa, Y., & Iida, T. (2009). Yo-yo intermittent recovery level 2 test in pubescent soccer players with relation to maturity category. *Football Science, 6*, 1–6.

McMillian, D. J., Moore, J. H., Hatler, B. S., & Taylor, D. C. (2006). Dynamic vs. static-stretching warm up: The effect on power and agility performance. *Journal of Strength and Conditioning Research, 20*(3), 492–499.

Newton, R. U., Gerber, A., Nimphius, S., Shim, J. K., et al. (2006). Determination of functional strength imbalance of the lower extremities. *Journal of Strength and Conditioning Research, 20*(4), 971–977.

Wiklander, J., & Lysholm, J. (1987). Simple tests for surveying muscle strength and muscle stiffness in sportsmen. *International Journal of Sports Medicine, 8*(1), 50–54.

■ CROSSOVER HOP TEST

Objective: Measure lower-body power

Age Range: High school to college age

Equipment Needed:

1. Open gym floor
2. Tape
3. Tape measure

Additional Personnel Needed: Test assistant

Setup:

1. A starting line is created on the floor (or a permanent line is utilized) (**Figure 7-9**).
2. A 15-centimeter (6-inch) blocked line is created on the floor.
3. The test assistant stands on the opposite side of the blocked line that the test performer begins behind.
4. The test performer may practice the protocol (described below).
5. The test performer stands behind the starting line and stands on one leg. If the test performer is balancing on the right leg, he or she should be on the right side of the blocked line. If he or she is balancing on the left leg, he or she should be on the left side of the blocked line.

Administration and Directions:

1. On the test administrator's "go" command, the test performer jumps forward and laterally on the balance leg. The test performer should jump over the blocked line (refer to Figure 7-9).
2. The test performer then lands on the opposite side of the blocked line on the balance foot.
3. The test performer then immediately jumps forward and laterally to the opposite side of the block line, landing on the balance foot.
4. The test performer then immediately jumps forward and laterally to the opposite side of the block line, landing on the balance foot.
5. After the third jump, the test performer balances on the landing foot for 2 seconds

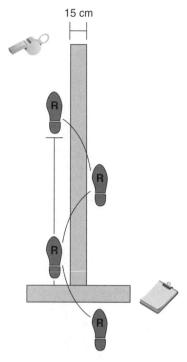

15 cm

Figure 7-9   Crossover Hop Test Setup and Administration

while the test assistant determines where the he or she landed.

6. The test performer's hops should be maximal.
7. Three trials are performed on each leg.

Scoring:

1. If the test performer loses his or her balance, or any other part of the body touches the ground besides the balance and hop leg, the trial is considered invalid and repeated. If this occurs several successive times, the test performer should rest before another attempt is given.
2. The distance from the starting line to the back of the test performer's *heel* is measured on each trial.
3. The farthest distance jumped by the test performer on each foot is recorded as the

final score. The total distance jumped on each foot may also be recorded as the final score.

Checklist: The test performer must

1. Not currently have a lower-body injury
2. Wear proper footwear for the surface the test is performed on
3. Have acceptable balance and coordination before this test is conducted
4. Begin and end the test while jumping on the same foot
5. Jumps directly forward on each attempt

References

Bandy, W. D., Rusche, K. R., & Tekulve, F. Y. (1994). Reliability and limb symmetry for five unilateral functional tests of the lower extremities. *Isokinetics and Exercise Science, 4*(3), 108–111.

Bolgla, L. A., & Keskula, D. R. (1997). Reliability of lower extremity functional performance tests. *Journal of Orthopaedic and Sports Physical Therapy, 26*(3), 138–142.

Noyes, F. R., Barber, S. D., & Mangine, R. E. (1991). Abnormal lower limb symmetry determined by function hop tests after anterior cruciate ligament rupture. *American Journal of Sports Medicine, 19*(5), 513–518.

Reid, A., Birmingham, T. B., Stratford, P. W., & Alcock, G. K. (2007). Hop testing provides a reliable and valid outcome measure during a rehabilitation after anterior cruciate ligament reconstruction. *Physical Therapy, 87*(3), 337–349.

Ross, M. D., Langford, B., & Whelan, P. J. (2002). Test-retest reliability of four single-leg horizontal hop tests. *Journal of Strength and Conditioning Research, 16*(4), 617–622.

Wilk, K. E., Romaniello, W. T., Soscia, S. M., Arrigo, C. A., & Andrews, J. A. (1994). The relationship between subjective knee scores, isokinetic testing, and functional testing in the ACL-reconstructed knee. *Journal of Orthopaedic and Sports Physical Therapy, 20*(2), 60–73.

■ 6-METER TIMED HOP TEST

Objective: Measure lower-leg horizontal power

Age Range: High school to college age

Equipment Needed:

1. Open grass field or gym floor
2. Stopwatch
3. Tape measure
4. Two cones

Additional Personnel Needed: Test assistant

Setup:

1. The two cones are placed 6 meters (19.5 feet) apart in a straight line (**Figure 7-10**).
2. The test assistant stands perpendicular to the starting line and starts the test performer on the course.
3. The test administrator stands perpendicular to the finish line and times the test performer.
4. The test performer may practice the test protocol (described below).
5. The test performer stands behind the starting line on one leg.

Administration and Directions:

1. On the test assistant's "go" command, the test performer jumps forward as fast as possible (utilizing only the balance leg) continuously until they cross the 6-meter line (refer to Figure 7-10).
2. The test performer should be encouraged to take large one-legged hops.
3. Three trials are performed on each leg.

Scoring:

1. If the test performer loses his or her balance or if any other part of the body touches the ground besides the balance and hop leg, the trial is considered invalid and must be repeated. If this occurs several successive times, the test performer should rest before making another attempt.

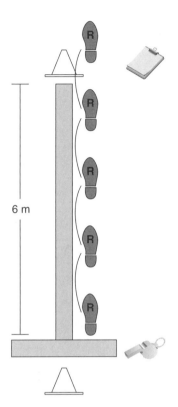

Figure 7-10   6-Meter Timed Hop Test Setup and Administration

2. The test administrator begins timing the trial on the test assistant's "go" command and stops timing the trial when the test performer's foot crosses the finish line.
3. The final score can be recorded as the fastest time on each foot or the average of all the times on each foot.

Checklist: The test performer must

1. Not currently have a lower-body injury
2. Wear proper footwear for the surface the test is performed on
3. Have acceptable balance and coordination before this test is conducted

4. Begin and end the test on the same foot
5. Jump directly forward on each attempt

References

Bandy, W. D., Rusche, K. R., & Tekulve, F. Y. (1994). Reliability and limb symmetry for five unilateral functional tests of the lower extremities. *Isokinetics and Exercise Science*, *4*(3), 108–111.

Bolgla, L. A., & Keskula, D. R. (1997). Reliability of lower extremity functional performance tests. *Journal of Orthopaedic and Sports Physical Therapy*, *26*(3), 138–142.

Booher, L. D., Hench, K. M., Worrell, T. W., & Stikeleather, J. (1993). Reliability of three single-leg hop tests. *Journal of Sport Rehabilitation*, *2*, 165–170.

Noyes, F. R., Barber, S. D., & Mangine, R. E. (1991). Abnormal lower limb symmetry determined by function hop tests after anterior cruciate ligament rupture. *American Journal of Sports Medicine*, *19*(5), 513–518.

Reid, A., Birmingham, T. B., Stratford, P. W., & Alcock, G. K. (2007). Hop testing provides a reliable and valid outcome measure during a rehabilitation after anterior cruciate ligament reconstruction. *Physical Therapy*, *87*(3), 337–349.

Ross, M. D., Langford, B., & Whelan, P. J. (2002). Test-retest reliability of four single-leg horizontal hop tests. *Journal of Strength and Conditioning Research*, *16*(4), 617–622.

Wilk, K. E., Romaniello, W. T., Soscia, S. M., Arrigo, C. A., & Andrews, J. A. (1994). The relationship between subjective knee scores, isokinetic testing, and functional testing in the ACL-reconstructed knee. *Journal of Orthopaedic and Sports Physical Therapy*, *20*(2), 60–73.

■ SQUARE HOP TEST

Objective: Measure lower-leg power and endurance

Age Range: High school to college age

Equipment Needed:

1. Flat gym floor
2. Tape
3. Tape measure
4. Stopwatch

Additional Personnel Needed: Test assistant

Setup:

1. A 40- by 40-centimeter (15- by 15-inch) square is created with tape on the floor with an X in the center of the square. This is the inner square (**Figure 7-11**).

2. Another square 10 centimeters (4 inches) is created outside the first square. This is the outer square.

3. The test administrator and test assistant should stand on opposite sides of the squares.

4. The test performer places the hands behind the back and stands on the X with one foot. The foot the test performer stands on determines the direction he or she will jump (described as follows).

5. The test performer may practice the protocol (described as follows) at partial speed.

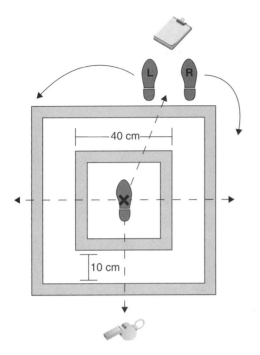

Figure 7-11 Square Hop Test Setup and Administration

Administration and Directions:

1. On the test administrator's "go" command, the test performer jumps from the X *beyond* the outer square and back to the X as many times as possible in 30 seconds (refer to Figure 7-11).
2. If the test performer is balancing on the *right leg*, he or she should jump in a *clockwise* direction.
3. If the test performer is balancing on the *left leg*, he or she should jump in a *counter-clockwise* direction.
4. The test performer does not need to jump directly back onto the X when returning to the inner square, but he or she should be encouraged to jump near the X, because the farther away he or she is from the X makes the next jump more difficult to complete.

5. No part of the test performer's foot may touch the lines that designate the inner or outer squares during this test (jump error).
6. If a jump error occurs, or if balance is lost during the trial, the test performer should regain the correct position and continue the trial. The test administrator should not stop the time.
7. One trial is performed on each leg.

Scoring:

1. The test assistant counts the number of times the test performer jumps in 30 seconds.
2. The test administrator counts the number of successful jumps the test performer completes in 30 seconds. A successful jump is when the test performer jumps from the inner square to beyond the outer square in the correct direction. The test performer's foot must be completely outside the outer square and inside the inner square to count as a successful jump.
3. The number of successful jumps is divided by the number of jump attempts.

successful jumps ÷ jump attempts

4. If more than 25% of the jump attempts result in errors, the test performer should be given a 3-minute rest before attempting another trial for that foot.
5. The number of successful jumps is recorded as the final score.

Checklist: The test performer must

1. Not currently have a lower-body injury
2. Have adequate balance before this test is performed
3. Keep the hands behind the back during this test
4. Understand he or she should not touch any of the square lines
5. Jump in the correct direction based on the balance leg

References

Gustavsson, A., Neeter, C., Thomee, P., et al. (2006). A test battery for evaluating hop performance in patients with an ACL injury and patients who have undergone ACL reconstruction. *Knee Surgery, Sports Traumatology, Arthroscopy, 14*, 778–788.

Ostenberg, A., Roos, E., Ekdahl, C., & Roos, H. (1998). Isokinetic knee extensor strength and functional performance in healthy female soccer players. *Scandinavian Journal of Medicine and Science in Sports, 8*, 257–264.

■ SIDE HOP TEST

Objective: Measure lower-leg power and endurance

Age Range: High school to college age

Equipment Needed:

1. Flat gym floor
2. Tape
3. Tape measure
4. Stopwatch

Additional Personnel Needed: Test assistant

Setup:

1. Two parallel lines are created on the floor 40 centimeters (15 inches) apart (**Figure 7-12**).

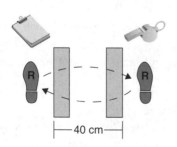

Figure 7-12 Side Hop Test Setup and Administration

2. The test administrator and test assistant should stand on opposite lines, perpendicular to the line.
3. The test performer places his or her hands behind the back and stands behind the line on one foot.
4. The test performer may practice the protocol (described below) at partial speed.

Administration and Directions:

1. On the test administrator's "go" command, the test performer jumps from the line he or she is standing behind to *beyond* the opposite line as many times as possible in 30 seconds (refer to Figure 7-12).
2. No part of the test performer's foot may touch the lines (jump error).
3. If a jump error occurs or the test performer loses his or her balance during the trial, the test performer should regain the correct position and continue the trial. The test administrator should not stop the time.
4. One trial is performed on each leg.

Scoring:

1. The test assistant counts the number of times the test performer jumps in 30 seconds.
2. The test administrator counts the number of successful jumps the test performer

completes in 30 seconds going toward the opposite line. A successful jump is when the test performer jumps beyond the line that the test performer is moving toward. The test performer's foot must be completely beyond the line to count as a successful jump.

3. The number of successful jumps is divided by the number of jump attempts.

successful jumps ÷ jump attempts

4. If more than 25% of the jump attempts result in errors, the test performer should be given a 3-minute rest before attempting another trial for that foot.
5. The number of successful jumps is recorded as the final score.

Checklist: The test performer must

1. Not currently have a lower-body injury
2. Have adequate balance before this test is performed

3. Keep the hands behind the back during this test
4. Understand he or she should not touch any of the lines

References

Gustavsson, A., Neeter, C., Thomee, P., et al. (2006). A test battery for evaluating hop performance in patients with an ACL injury and patients who have undergone ACL reconstruction. *Knee Surgery, Sports Traumatology, Arthroscopy, 14,* 778–788.

Itoh, H., Kurosaka, M., Yoshiya, S., Ichihashi, N., & Mizuno, K. (1998). Evaluation of functional deficits determined by four different hop tests in patients with anterior cruciate ligament deficiency. *Knee Surgery, Sports Traumatology, Arthroscopy, 6,* 241–245.

■ HOP AND STOP TEST

Also Known as: Hop, Stop, and Leap Test

Objective: Evaluate force production and force absorption of the lower extremities and identify muscular and balance asymmetries between right and left legs; this test may be utilized to evaluate the risk an individual has of sustaining an ACL injury

Age Range: High school to college age

Equipment Needed:

1. Stopwatch
2. Open gym or outdoor surface
3. Tape or cone
4. Tape measure

Additional Personnel Needed: One or two test assistants

Setup:

1. The test performer's height is measured.
2. A starting line is designated by tape, cone, or a permanent line.
3. The test performer stands behind the starting line.
4. The test performer balances on one foot, places the hands on the hips, bends the non-balance knee to 90°, and flexes the non-balance hip to 90°. The non-balance knee should be approximately the height

of the navel. All tests begin from this starting position (**Figure 7-13**).

5. The test performer may practice the test procedure (described below) at a minimum effort.

Administration and Directions: This test is separated into two tests: hop test and leap test.

1. Hop test (**Figure 7-14**): Evaluating force production
   a. On the test administrator's "go" command, the test performer maintains the starting position, bends the balance leg, and hops forward as far as possible.
   b. The test performer lands on the balance leg (i.e., if the test performer balances on the right leg, he or she should land on the right leg).

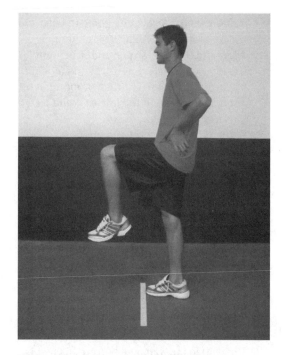

Figure 7-13   Hop and Stop Test Starting Position

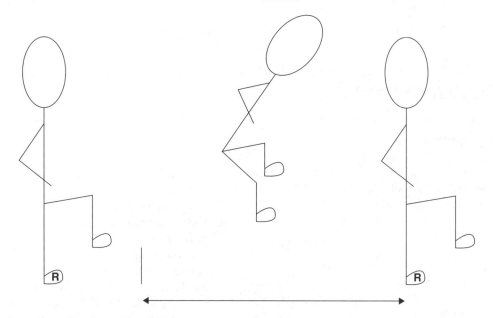

Figure 7-14   Hop Test Administration

c. The test assistant marks where the back of the test performer's *heel* lands.

d. Three successful trials are performed on each foot.

2. Leap test (**Figure 7-15**): Evaluating force absorption

   a. On the test administrator's "go" command, the test performer maintains the starting position, bends the balance leg, and hops forward as far as possible.

   b. The test performer lands on the non-balance leg (i.e., if the test performer balances on the right leg, he or she should land on the left leg).

   c. Once the test performer lands, he or she must completely stop and maintain a one-leg balance position within one second of landing before the trial is considered successful. The test performer must demonstrate body control (i.e., be properly balanced).

   d. After the test performer has stabilized him- or herself within 1 second, the test assistant marks where the back of the test performer's *heel* lands.

   e. Three successful trials are performed on each foot.

3. If any of the following occur during the execution of either test, the trial is stopped, considered invalid, and restarted:

   a. The test performer drops the non-balance leg during the jumping motion (**Figure 7-16**).

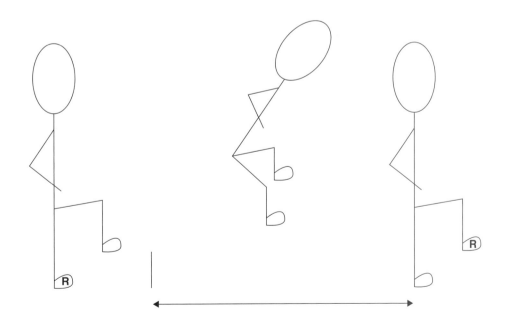

Figure 7-15 Leap Test Administration

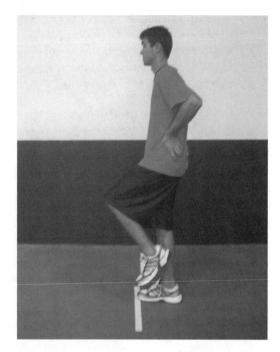

Figure 7-16 Hop and Stop Test Incorrect Administration

   b. The test performer removes the hands from the hips during the test.

4. If a test performer is having difficulty completing either test and needs more than five trials on a particular leg, he or she should be given a 2-minute rest period before more trials are attempted.

Scoring:

1. Hop test
   a. The distance from the back of the test performer's *heel* to the starting line is measured on each foot for each trial

(a total of six measurements) and then averaged for each foot.
   b. A test performer passes the hop test if the hop is *at least* 89% of his or her height. Each leg is evaluated separately. A score of less than 89% indicates the test performer should work on force production for that leg.

2. Leap test
   a. The distance from the back of the test performer's *heel* to the starting line is measured on each foot for each trial (a total of six measurements) and then averaged for each foot.
   b. A test performer passes the leap test if the leap is *at least* 109% of his or her height. Each leg is evaluated separately. A score of less than 109% indicates the test performer should work on force absorption for the landing leg.

Checklist: The test performer must

1. Not currently have a lower-body injury
2. Wear proper footwear for the surface the test is performed on
3. Maintain proper form during the execution of the test

References

Boone, J., & Cook, G. (2006, October). Best foot forward. *Training and Conditioning*, 37–42.

Juris, P. M., Phillips, E. M., Dalpe, C., Edwards, C., Gotlin, R. S., & Kane, D. J. (1997). A dynamic test of lower extremity function following anterior cruciate ligament reconstruction and rehabilitation. *Journal of Orthopedic and Sports Physical Therapy, 26*(4), 184–194.

■ SEATED MEDICINE BALL THROW TEST

Objective: Measure upper-body power

Age Range: High school to college age

Equipment Needed:

1. Tape measure
2. Adjustable bench or chair with a back support (with ankle pads at the base if available)
3. Straps
4. Five- or 11-pound (2.2- or 5-kilogram) medicine ball
5. Open gym floor with no hanging objects that can be struck

Additional Personnel Needed: Test assistant

Setup:

1. The test performer sits on the bench (**Figure 7-17**).

2. The test performer is secured to the back support to minimize the involvement of the trunk and leg musculature during the test.
3. The test assistant is positioned away from the bench to determine where the medicine ball lands.
4. The test performer is given a medicine ball and places it in the lap. The same-weight medicine ball should be utilized for all trials.

Administration and Directions:

1. On the test administrator's "go" command, the test performer brings the medicine ball to the chest (**Figure 7-18**).
2. The test performer then pushes the medicine ball upward and outward at a

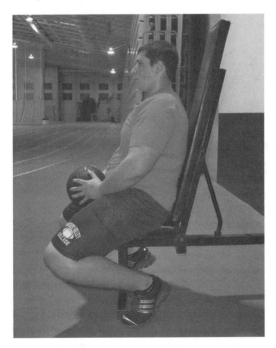

Figure 7-17   Seated Medicine Ball Throw Test Setup

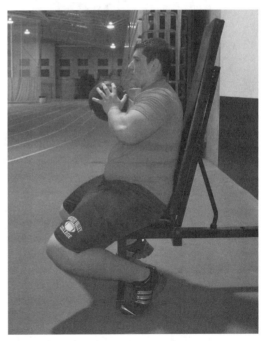

Figure 7-18   Seated Medicine Ball Throw Test Starting Position

45° angle using a technique similar to a basketball chest pass (**Figure 7-19**).

3. The test performer is given a 2-minute rest.
4. Three trials are performed.

Scoring:

1. The weight of the medicine ball should be documented.
2. The distance of each trial is measured from the base of the bench to where the medicine ball *lands* on the floor.
3. The best distance is recorded as the final score.

Checklist: The test performer must

1. Not currently have an upper-body injury
2. Be securely strapped to the bench

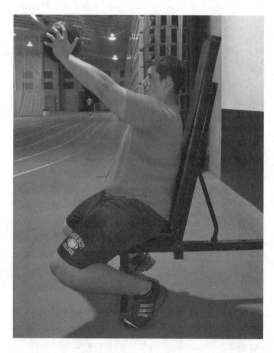

Figure 7-19   Seated Medicine Ball Throw Test Ending Position

3. Bring the medicine ball up to the chest and toss it quickly
4. Rest for 2 minutes between trials

References

Borrie, A., Mullan, N., & Palmer, C. (1998). The development of a medicine ball throw test for the assessment of upper body performance. *Journal of Sports Sciences, 16*(1), 38.

Cronin, J. B., & Owen, G. J. (2004). Upper-body strength and power assessment in women using a chest pass. *Journal of Strength and Conditioning Research, 18*(3), 401–404.

Falvo, M. J., Schilling, B. K., & Weiss, L. W. (2006). Techniques and considerations for determining isoinertial upper-body power. *Sports Biomechanics, 5*(2), 293–311.

Gore, C. J. (2000). *Physiological tests for elite athletes.* Australian Sports Commission. Champaign, IL: Human Kinetics.

Johnson, B. L., & Nelson, J. K. (1986). *Practical measurements for evaluation in physical education* (4th ed.). New York: MacMillan.

Nash, A. (2008, Fall). Seated medicine ball toss as a predictor of upper-body strength in untrained women. *Kentucky Newsletter for Health, Physical Education, Recreation, and Dance,* 27–30.

Sayers, A., Eveland Sayers, B., & Binkley, B. (2008). Preseason fitness testing in National Collegiate Athletic Association soccer. *Strength and Conditioning Journal, 30*(4), 70–75.

Semenick, D. (1984). Anaerobic testing: Practical applications. *National Strength and Conditioning Association Journal, 6*(5), 45, 70–73.

Vossen, J. F., Kramer, J. F., Gurke, D. G., & Vossen, D. P. (2000). Comparison of dynamic push-up training and plyometric push-up training on upper-body power and strength. *Journal of Strength and Conditioning Research, 14*(3), 248–253.

■ SEATED SHOT PUT TEST

Objective: Measure upper-body power

Age Range: High school to college age

Equipment Needed:

1. Tape measure
2. Adjustable bench or chair with a back support and ankle pads at the base (if available)
3. Straps
4. Standard 10-pound (4.5-kilogram) indoor shot put
5. Open gym floor (with a mat protecting the floor), a long jump pit, or a similar area

Additional Personnel Needed: Test assistant

Setup:

1. The test performer sits on the bench or chair (**Figure 7-20**).

2. The test performer's ankles are placed behind the ankle pads or otherwise secured to the chair, minimizing the involvement of the trunk and leg musculature during the test.
3. The test assistant is positioned away from the bench to determine where the shot put lands.
4. The test performer is given a shot put and places it in the lap.

Administration and Directions:

1. On the test administrator's "go" command, the test performer brings the shot put to the chest, holding it with both hands, keeping the forearms parallel to the ground (**Figure 7-21**).

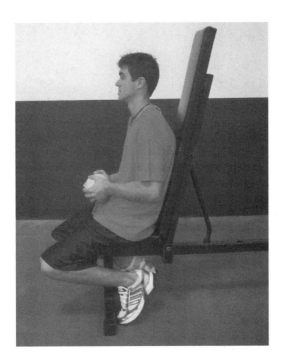

Figure 7-20   Seated Shot Put Test Setup

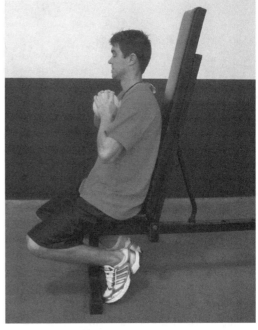

Figure 7-21   Seated Shot Put Test Starting Position

2. The test performer then pushes the shot put away from the body using a technique similar to a basketball chest pass (**Figure 7-22**).

3. The test performer is given a 2-minute rest.

4. Three trials are performed.

Scoring:

1. The distance of each trial is measured from the base of the bench or chair to where the shot put *lands* on the floor.

2. The best distance is recorded as the final score.

Checklist: The test performer must

1. Not currently have an upper-body injury
2. Be securely strapped to the bench or chair

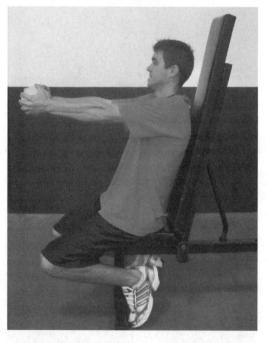

Figure 7-22 Seated Shot Put Test Ending Position

3. Bring the shot put to the chest and toss it quickly

4. Rest for 2 minutes between trials

References

Coaches roundtable: Testing for football. (1983). *National Strength and Conditioning Association Journal, 5*(5), 12–19.

Falvo, M. J., Schilling, B. K., & Weiss, L. W. (2006). Techniques and considerations for determining isoinertial upper-body power. *Sports Biomechanics, 5*(2), 293–311.

Gillespie, J., & Keenum, S. (1987). A validity and reliability analysis of the seated shot put as a test of power. *Journal of Human Movement Studies, 13*(2), 97–105.

Gore, C. J. (2000). *Physiological tests for elite athletes.* Australian Sports Commission. Champaign, IL: Human Kinetics.

Mayhew, J. L., Bemben, M. G., & Rohrs, D. M. (1992). Seated shot put as a measure of upper body power in adolescent wrestlers. *Pediatric Exercise Science, 4*, 78–84.

Mayhew, J. L., Bemben, M. G., Piper, F. C., Ware, J. S., et al. (1993). Assessing bench press power in college football players: The seated shot put. *Journal of Strength and Conditioning Research, 7*(2), 95–100.

Mayhew, J. L., Bemben, M. G., Rohrs, D. M., Piper, F. C., & Willman, M. K. (1995). Comparison of upper body power in adolescent wrestlers and basketball players. *Pediatric Exercise Science, 7*, 422–431.

Mayhew, J. L., Bemben, M. G., Rohrs, D. M., Ware, J., & Bemben, D. A. (1991). Seated shot put as a measure of upper body power in college males. *Journal of Human Movement Studies, 21*(3), 137–148.

■ STANDING MEDICINE BALL CHEST PASS TEST

Objective: Measure upper-body power

Age Range: Middle school to adult

Equipment Needed:

1. Open gym floor or similar surface
2. Tape (a permanent solid line can be utilized)
3. Tape measure
4. Five- or 11-pound (2.2- or 5-kilogram) medicine ball

Additional Personnel Needed: Test assistant

Setup:

1. A solid line is created on the floor (or a permanent solid line is selected). The test assistant is positioned away from the line where the test performer will throw the medicine ball.
2. The test performer is given a medicine ball.
3. The test performer holds the medicine ball against the abdomen with the arms relaxed (**Figure 7-23**).
4. The test performer faces the direction where the medicine ball will be thrown and places both feet directly behind the line.

Administration and Directions:

1. On the test administrator's "go" command, the test performer brings the medicine ball to the chest, holding it with both hands, keeping the forearms parallel to the floor (**Figure 7-24**).
2. The test performer then immediately pushes the medicine ball away from the body using a technique similar to a basketball chest pass (**Figure 7-25**).
3. The test performer is given a 2-minute rest.
4. Three trials are performed.

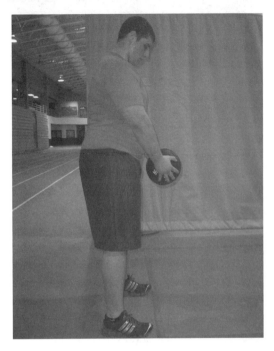

Figure 7-23 Standing Medicine Ball Chest Pass Test Setup

Scoring:

1. The weight of the medicine ball should be documented.
2. The distance of each trial is measured from the starting line to where the medicine ball *lands* on the floor.
3. The best distance is recorded as the final score.

Checklist: The test performer must

1. Not currently have an upper-body injury
2. Keep the entire body behind the line while throwing the medicine ball

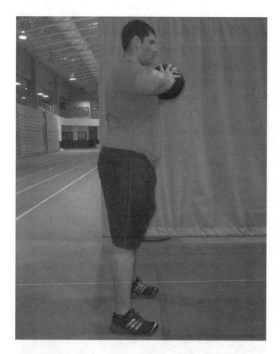

Figure 7-24 Standing Medicine Ball Chest Pass Test Starting Position

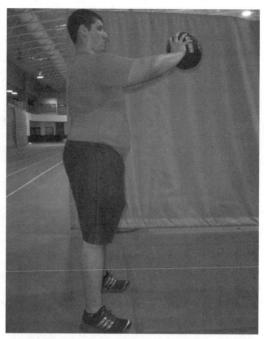

Figure 7-25 Standing Medicine Ball Chest Pass Test Ending Position

3. Bring the medicine ball to the chest and toss it quickly
4. Not flex the abdomen forward or backward during the passing movement
5. Rest for 2 minutes between trials

References

Falvo, M. J., Schilling, B. K., & Weiss, L. W. (2006). Techniques and considerations for determining isoinertial upper-body power. *Sports Biomechanics, 5*(2), 293–311.

Salonia, M. A., Chu, D. A., Cheifetz, P. M., & Freidhoff, G. C. (2004). Upper-body power as measured by medicine-ball throw distance and its relationship to class level among 10- and 11-year-old female participants in club gymnastics. *Journal of Strength and Conditioning Research, 18*(4), 695–702.

■ STANDING MEDICINE BALL THROW TEST

Objective: Measure upper-body and abdominal power

Age Range: Middle school to adult

Equipment Needed:

1. Open gym floor or similar surface
2. Tape (a permanent solid line can be utilized)
3. Tape measure
4. Five- or 11-pound (2.2- or 5-kilogram) medicine ball

Additional Personnel Needed: Test assistant

Setup:

1. A solid line is created on the floor (or a permanent solid line is selected). The test assistant is positioned away from the line where the test performer will throw the medicine ball (**Figure 7-26**).
2. The test performer is given a medicine ball.
3. The test performer holds the medicine ball with both hands and places the medicine ball behind the head.
4. The test performer faces the direction where the medicine ball will be thrown and places one foot directly behind the line. The test performer takes one step back with the opposite foot.

Administration and Directions:

1. On the test administrator's "go" command, the test performer brings the back foot towards the line (**Figure 7-27**).

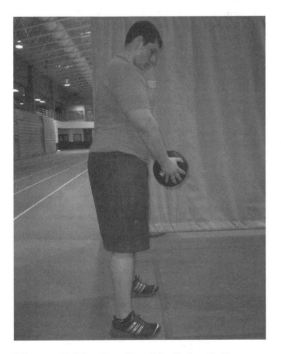

Figure 7-26 Standing Medicine Ball Throw Test Setup

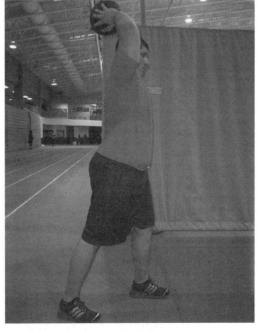

Figure 7-27 Standing Medicine Ball Throw Test Starting Position

2. The test performer then throws the medicine ball over the head in the same motion similar to a soccer throw-in (**Figure 7-28**).
3. The throwing motion should not carry the test performer over the starting line until after the medicine ball lands.
4. The test performer receives a 2-minute rest.
5. Three trials are performed.

Scoring:

1. The weight of the medicine ball should be documented.

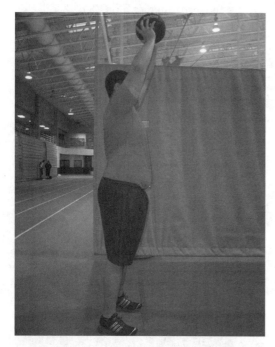

Figure 7-28 Standing Medicine Ball Throw Test Ending Position

2. The distance of each trial is measured from the line to where the medicine ball *lands* on the floor.
3. The best distance is recorded as the final score.

Checklist: The test performer must

1. Not currently have an upper-body injury before performing this test
2. Keep the entire body and toes behind the line while throwing the ball and immediately afterward
3. Throw the medicine ball directly over the head

References

Falvo, M. J., Schilling, B. K., & Weiss, L. W. (2006). Techniques and considerations for determining isoinertial upper-body power. *Sports Biomechanics, 5*(2), 293–311.

Gabbett, T., & Georgieff, B. (2007). Physiological and anthropometric characteristics of Australian junior national, state, and novice volleyball players. *Journal of Strength and Conditioning Research, 21*(3), 902–908.

Roetert, E. P., Brown, S. W., Piorkowski, P. A., & Woods, R. B. (1996). Fitness comparisons among three different levels of elite tennis players. *Journal of Strength and Conditioning Research, 10*(3), 139–143.

Salonia, M. A., Chu, D. A., Cheifetz, P. M., & Freidhoff, G. C. (2004). Upper-body power as measured by medicine-ball throw distance and its relationship to class level among 10- and 11-year-old female participants in club gymnastics. *Journal of Strength and Conditioning Research, 18*(4), 695–702.

■ BACKWARD OVERHEAD MEDICINE BALL THROW TEST

Objective: Measure total body power

Age Range: Middle school to adult

Equipment Needed:

1. Open gym floor with a high ceiling, open field, or similar surface
2. Tape, cone, or a permanent solid line
3. Tape measure
4. Five- or 11-pound (2.2- or 5-kilogram) medicine ball

Additional Personnel Needed: Test assistant

Setup:

1. A starting line is created with tape or a cone, or a permanent solid line is selected. The test assistant is positioned away from the line where the test

performer will throw the medicine ball (**Figure 7-29**).

2. The test performer holds the medicine ball with both hands, thumbs pointing upward, and arms relaxed.
3. The test performer turns his or her back toward the direction the medicine ball will be thrown and places the heels on the starting line.

Administration and Directions:

1. On the test administrator's "go" command, the test performer bends the knees, flexes the hips, knees, and trunk, and lowers the medicine ball just below the hips (**Figure 7-30**).

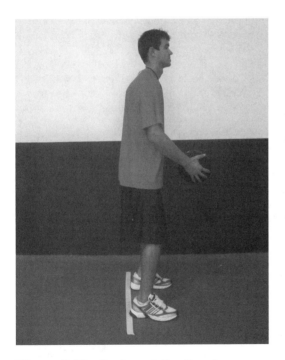

Figure 7-29   Backward Overhead
Medicine Ball Throw Test Setup

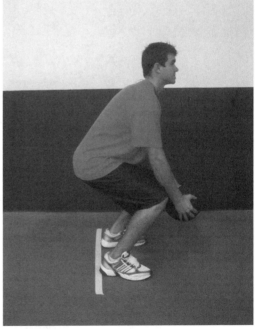

Figure 7-30   Backward Overhead
Medicine Ball Throw Test Starting Position

2. The test performer then rapidly springs upward and tosses the medicine ball toward the measurement area in the same motion (**Figure 7-31**).

3. The test performer's feet may leave the ground as the medicine ball is released, but momentum should not carry him or her over the starting line.

4. The test performer is given a 2-minute rest.

5. Three trials are performed.

Scoring:

1. The weight of the medicine ball should be documented.

2. The distance of each trial is measured from the line to where the medicine ball *lands.*

3. The best distance is recorded as the final score.

Checklist: The test performer must

1. Not currently have an upper- or lower-body injury

2. Keep the entire body and toes behind the line while throwing the medicine ball

3. Go quickly from the starting position to the finishing position

4. Throw the medicine ball outward, not upward

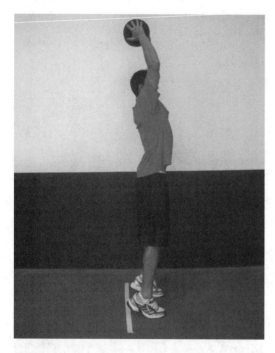

Figure 7-31 Backward Overhead Medicine Ball Throw Test Ending Position

References

Mayhew, J. L., Bird, M., Cole, M. L., Kock, A. J., et al. (2005). Comparison of the backward overhead medicine ball throw to power production in college football players. *Journal of Strength and Conditioning Research, 19*(3), 514–518.

Roetert, E. P., Brown, S. W., Piorkowski, P. A., & Woods, R. B. (1996). Fitness comparisons among three different levels of elite tennis players. *Journal of Strength and Conditioning Research, 10*(3), 139–143.

Salonia, M. A., Chu, D. A., Cheifetz, P. M., & Freidhoff, G. C. (2004). Upper-body power as measured by medicine-ball throw distance and its relationship to class level among 10- and 11-year-old female participants in club gymnastics. *Journal of Strength and Conditioning Research, 18*(4), 695–702.

Stockbrugger, B. A., & Haennel, R. G. (2001). Validity and reliability of a medicine ball explosive power test. *Journal of Strength and Conditioning Research, 15*(4), 431–438.

CHAPTER

8

Aerobic Capacity and Cardiorespiratory Fitness Testing

Cardiorespiratory fitness, also termed aerobic capacity or aerobic power, is the body's ability to perform moderate to high-intensity physical activity for extended durations. Cardiorespiratory fitness can also be thought of as the maximum rate at which an individual can produce energy from the oxidation of carbohydrates and fats. Cardiorespiratory fitness requires the interaction of the heart, lungs, blood, arteries, veins, capillaries, and muscle cells working together to adjust to vigorous and prolonged exercise and recover from the exercise. Generally, individuals who attain good scores on cardiorespiratory fitness tests can perform the same amount of work, while expending less energy to perform that work, than an individual who scores lower.

The test administrator should ensure the test performer is in good general health before undergoing cardiorespiratory fitness testing. If there is any doubt, the test performer should undergo a physical exam and bring documentation of proper general health before cardiovascular fitness testing is conducted. The test performer should warm up and stretch without expending substantial energy before engaging in cardiovascular fitness tests. Having the test performer complete the requirements of the cardiovascular fitness test at a lower intensity and pace should be an adequate warm-up. The test performer should be instructed in proper cardiovascular fitness testing principles, particularly the concept that he or she should not start the test at an unsustainable (fast) pace. The test performer should perform the test in a controlled and consistent manner. Additionally, each test performer needs to perform at his or her individual best and should not participate in a group during the test. Cardiorespiratory fitness testing should be performed as the final test in a test battery (that day). Balance, agility, speed, strength, and lower-extremity local muscular endurance tests administered after a cardio-vascular fitness test may result in poor scores.

Typically in research, cardiovascular fitness test results are expressed as (converted to) a VO_{2max}.

■ COOPER TEST: 9-MINUTE OR 12-MINUTE WALK/RUN TEST

Objective: Measure cardiorespiratory fitness

Age Range: 5 to college age (9-minute run) *or* junior high to adult (12-minute run)

Equipment Needed:

1. Stopwatch
2. Whistle
3. Flat, measured running surface with no sharp turns that can be observed by the test administrator
4. Multiple course markers (i.e., cones)
5. Lap counter or paper and pencil

Additional Personnel Needed: One or two test assistants

Setup:

1. Measure and mark the course in a consistent manner (i.e., every 10 to 25 yards, or 9 to 22 meters). The test administrator should be able to quickly determine how far each test performer has traveled. The distance of the entire course (lap) should be known.
2. Explain to the test performer the benefits of maintaining a constant pace and not starting too fast. Multiple test performers should not run in a group while conducting this test. Each test performer must give his or her best effort.
3. The test administrator explains to the test performer what constitutes the designated course.

4. If multiple test performers are being evaluated simultaneously, multiple test assistants may be necessary to assist the test administrator document/count the laps completed by each test performer.
5. The test performer lines up behind the starting line.

Administration and Directions:

1. On the test administrator's "go" command, the test performer runs the designated course.
2. The test performer runs the course continuously until the test administrator stops the test.
3. The test performer may walk during this test, but should only do so sporadically to recover. The test performer should be encouraged to jog when he or she has recovered.
4. When the test administrator gives the "stop" command (after either 9 or 12 minutes), the test performer stops where he or she is on the course until the position can be properly documented by the test administrator or a test assistant.
5. After the test performer's location is documented, he or she should cool down.
6. One trial is performed.

Scoring:

1. The total distance traveled by each test performer is measured to the nearest 10 yards (9 meters). This is best achieved by counting the number of laps multiplied by the length of the course and adding the distance of any partial lap.
2. It is essential to properly measure, mark, and record the length of each partial lap completed as well as count the number of laps completed, to determine the test performer's score.
3. The distance traveled is recorded as the final score.
4. The distance traveled can be utilized to determine the relative fitness level of the test performer.

Distance (Miles)	Fitness Level
<1.0	Very poor
1.0 to 1.24	Poor
1.25 to 1.49	Fair
1.50 to 1.74	Good
>1.75	Excellent

5. The 9-minute run test can be converted into a VO_{2max} figure:

$$VO_{2max} = (0.024 \times \text{run distance in yards}) - 4.7$$

6. The 12-minute run test can be converted into a VO_{2max} figure:

$$VO_{2max} = (\text{distance in miles} - 0.3138) \div 0.0278$$

Checklist: The test performer must

1. Know what constitutes the course
2. Understand how to perform a long-distance run
3. Not perform this test in a group
4. Stop when the test administrator signals the end of the test and remain in place until his or her position is properly documented

References

American Association for Health, Physical Education, Recreation, and Dance. (1980). *Lifetime health related physical fitness.* Reston, VA: AAHPERD.

American College of Sports Medicine. (2006). *ACSM's guidelines for exercise testing and prescription* (7th ed.). Philadelphia: Lippincott Williams & Wilkins.

Arabas, J. L., Peters Anderson, M. M. E., Arabas, J. R., Arabas, C. D., & Mayhew, J. L. (1996). Estimation of VO_{2max} from 9-minute run performance. *IAHPERD Journal, 29*(2).

Baechle, T. R., & Earle, R. W. (2008). *Essentials of strength training and conditioning* (3rd ed.). Champaign, IL: Human Kinetics.

Brodie, D. A. (1996). *A reference manual for human performance measurement in the field of physical education and sports sciences.* Lewiston, NY: Edwin Mellen Press.

Calders, P., Deforche, B., Verschelde, S., Bouckaert, J., et al. (2008). Predictors of 6-minute walk test and 12-minute walk/run test in obese children and adolescents. *European Journal of Pediatrics, 167,* 563–568.

Cooper, K. H. (1968). A means of assessing maximal oxygen intake. *JAMA, 203*(3), 135–138.

Doolittle, T. L., & Bigbee, R. (1968). The twelve-minute run-walk: A test of cardiorespiratory fitness of adolescent boys. *Research Quarterly, 39*(3), 491–495.

Drowatzky, K. L., & Anders, F. F. (1996). Comparison of the Rockport walking and Cooper walk-run fitness tests. *Clinical Kinesiology, 50*(2), 36–39.

Heyward, V. H. (2006). *Advanced fitness assessment and exercise prescription* (5th ed.). Champaign, IL: Human Kinetics.

Johnson, B. L., & Nelson, J. K. (1986). *Practical measurements for evaluation in physical education* (4th ed.). New York: MacMillan.

Maksud, M. G., & Coutts, K. D. (1971). Application of the Cooper twelve-minute run-walk test to young males. *Research Quarterly, 42*(1), 54–59.

McNaughton, L., Hall, P., & Cooley, D. (1998). Validation of several methods of estimating maximal oxygen uptake in young men. *Perceptual and Motor Skills*, *87*, 575–584.

Prentice, W. E. (1997). *Fitness for college and life* (5th ed.). St. Louis: Mosby.

Rosch, D., Hodgson, R., Peterson, L., Graf-Baumann, T., Junge, A., Chomiak, J., & Dvorak, J. (2000). Assessment and evaluation of football performance. *American Journal of Sports Medicine*, *28*(5), S29–S49.

■ 1-MILE (1.6-KILOMETER) OR 1.5-MILE (2.4-KILOMETER) RUN/WALK TEST

Objective: Measure cardiorespiratory fitness

Age Range: 5 to adult (1-mile run) *or* 13 to adult (1.5-mile run)

Equipment Needed:

1. Stopwatch
2. Flat, measured running surface with no sharp turns
3. Calibrated scale and tape measure (if VO_{2max} is calculated)

Additional Personnel Needed: One or two test assistants

Setup:

1. The test administrator explains to the test performer(s) the benefits of maintaining a constant pace and not starting too fast. Multiple test performers should not run in a group during this test. Each test performer must give his or her best effort.
2. The test administrator explains to the test performer(s) what constitutes the designated course.
3. If multiple test performers are being evaluated simultaneously, multiple test assistants may be necessary to assist the test administrator document/count the laps completed by each test performer.

4. The test performer lines up behind the starting line.

Administration and Directions:

1. On the test administrator's "go" signal, the test performer runs the designated course as fast as possible.
2. The test performer may walk during this test, but should only do so sporadically to recover. The test performer should be encouraged to jog once he or she has recovered.
3. One trial is performed.

Scoring:

1. The test administrator documents the time each test performer finishes the course in minutes and seconds.
2. If multiple test performers are tested simultaneously, multiple test assistants may be necessary to assist the test administrator in determining the place each test performer finishes and the corresponding time.
3. The time is recorded as the final score.
4. The 1-mile run test can be converted into a VO_{2max} figure by first determining body mass index (BMI). (Gender: male = 1;

female = 0. Time in minutes and seconds: seconds are divided by 60. For example, 13 minutes and 40 seconds is converted to 13.66.)

$$BMI = \text{weight in kilograms} \div (\text{height in meters})^2$$

$$VO_{2max} = -8.41(\text{1-mile run time in minutes}) + 0.34(\text{1-mile run time in minutes})^2 + 0.21(\text{age in years} \times \text{sex}) - 0.84(BMI)$$

5. The 1.5-mile run test can be converted into a VO_{2max} figure.

$$VO_{2max} = 3.5 + 483 \div (\text{1.5-mile run time in minutes})$$

Checklist: The test performer must

1. Complete the entire course and not take shortcuts
2. Not perform this test in a group

References

American Association for Health, Physical Education, Recreation, and Dance. (1980). *Lifetime health related physical fitness.* Reston, VA: AAHPERD.

American College of Sports Medicine. (2006). *ACSM's guidelines for exercise testing and prescription* (7th ed.). Philadelphia: Lippincott Williams & Wilkins.

Annesi, J. J., Westcott, W. L., Faigenbaum, A. D., & Unruh, J. L. (2005). Effects of a 12-week physical activity protocol delivered by YMCA after-school counselors (Youth Fit For Life) on fitness and self-efficacy changes in 5–12 year-old boys and girls. *Research Quarterly for Exercise and Sport, 76*(4), 468–476.

Baechle, T. R., & Earle, R. W. (2008). *Essentials of strength training and conditioning* (3rd ed.). Champaign, IL: Human Kinetics.

Castro-Pinero, J., Mora, J., Gonzalez-Montesinos, J. L., Sjostrom, M., & Ruiz, J. R. (2009). Criterion-related validity of the one-mile run/walk test in children aged 8–17 years. *Journal of Sports Sciences, 27*(4), 405–413.

Getchell, B., Mikesky, A. E., & Mikesky, K. N. (1998). *Physical fitness: A way of life* (5th ed.). Boston: Allyn and Bacon.

Heyward, V. H. (2006). *Advanced fitness assessment and exercise prescription* (5th ed.). Champaign, IL: Human Kinetics.

Johnson, B. L., & Nelson, J. K. (1986). *Practical measurements for evaluation in physical education* (4th ed.). New York: MacMillan.

Larsen, G. E., George, J. D., Alexander, J. L., Fellingham, G. W., Aldana, S. G., & Parcell, A. C. (2002). Prediction of maximum oxygen consumption from walking, jogging, or running. *Research Quarterly for Exercise and Sport, 73*(1), 66–72.

Mahar, M. T., Rowe, D. S., Parker, C. P., Mahar, F. J., Dawson, M., & Holt, J. E. (1997). Criterion-referenced and norm-referenced agreement between the mile run/walk and PACER. *Measurement in Physical Education and Exercise Science, 1*(4), 245–258.

McNaughton, L., Hall, P., & Cooley, D. (1998). Validation of several methods of estimating maximal oxygen uptake in young men. *Perceptual and Motor Skills, 87*, 575–584.

McSwegin, P., Pemberton, C., Petray, C., & Going, S. (1989). *Physical best: The AAHPERD guide to physical fitness education and assessment.* Reston, VA: AAHPERD.

Meredith, M. D., & Welk, C. J. *FITNESSGRAM®/ACTIVITYGRAM® test administration manual* (4th ed.). Champaign, IL: Human Kinetics.

Safrit, M. J. (1995). *Complete guide to youth fitness testing.* Champaign, IL: Human Kinetics.

Semenick, D. (1981). Conditioning program: Testing and evaluation. *National Strength and Conditioning Association Journal, 3*(2), 8–9.

Tritschler, K. (2000). *Barrow & McGee's practical measurement and assessment* (5th ed.). Philadelphia: Lippincott Williams & Wilkins.

■ SUBMAXIMAL MILE (1.6-KILOMETER) TRACK JOG TEST

Objective: Measure cardiorespiratory fitness from a submaximal exercise

Age Range: High school to adult

Equipment Needed:

1. An outdoor track is best. Any measured running surface 1 mile (1.6 kilometers) in length with no sharp turns is sufficient.
2. Stopwatch (one per test performer)
3. Heart rate monitor (one per test performer)
4. Calibrated scale

Additional Personnel Needed: One test partner per test performer *and* one or two additional test assistants

Setup:

1. The test performer is weighed (BW) without shoes and with minimal clothing (in kilograms).
2. The test performer is given a heart rate monitor and paired with a test partner or a test assistant.
3. The test administrator explains the test protocol (described below) to the test performer.
4. The test performer may practice jogging at the correct pace for 2 to 3 minutes (described under administration of this test).
5. The test performer may perform this test while running in a group as long as the proper pace is maintained.
6. The test performer lines up behind the starting line.

Administration and Directions:

1. On the test administrator's "go" command, the test performer runs around the designated course at the correct pace.

a. Men: May *not* run the mile (1.6 kilometers) faster than 8 minutes and should *not* complete a 440-yard (400-meter) lap faster than 2 minutes.

b. Women: May *not* run the mile (1.6 kilometers) faster than 9 minutes and should *not* complete a 440-yard (400-meter) lap faster than 2 minutes and 15 seconds (2.25 minutes).

c. Final exercise heart rate should *not* exceed 180 beats per minute (BPM).

2. The test performer should maintain a steady pace at all times and *not* sprint, especially at the end of the final lap.
3. It is the responsibility of the test partner and/or the test assistant to keep the test performer on the correct pace by informing the performer of the lap times.
4. One trial is performed.

Scoring:

1. If a heart rate monitor is utilized, the test administrator documents the test performer's exercise heart rate (EHR) when he or she crosses the finish line.
2. If a heart rate monitor is not utilized, the test assistant or test partner obtains the test performer's carotid pulse for 10 seconds, then multiplies that number by 6 to calculate the test performer's approximate heart rate. It is important to begin measuring the test performer's heart rate within 5 seconds after finishing the test.
3. The test administrator records the test performer's final mile jog time (MJT).
4. EHR, BW, and MJT are put into a formula to determine the VO_{2max}. (Time in minutes and seconds: seconds are divided by 60.

For example, 7 minutes and 00 seconds is converted to 7.33.)

$$\text{Men: VO}_{2max} = 108.844 - 0.1636(BW)$$
$$- 1.438(MJT)$$
$$- 0.1938(EHR)$$

$$\text{Women: VO}_{2max} = 100.5 - 0.1636(BW)$$
$$- 1.438(MJT)$$
$$- 0.1938(EHR)$$

5. The VO_{2max} calculation is recorded as the final score.

Checklist: The test performer must

1. Not sprint at any time during this test
2. Does not run faster than the maximal pace allowed

References

George, J. D., Vehrs, P. R., Allsen, P. E., Fellingham, G. W., & Fisher, A. G. VO_{2max} estimation from a submaximal 1-mile track jog for fit college-aged individuals. *Medicine and Science in Sports and Exercise, 25*(3), 401–406.

Tritschler, K. (2000). *Barrow & McGee's practical measurement and assessment* (5th ed.). Philadelphia: Lippincott Williams & Wilkins.

■ 1-MILE (1.6-KILOMETER) WALK TEST

Objective: Measure aerobic capacity; this test is an alternative to the PACER test

Age Range: 13 to adult

Equipment Needed:

1. Stopwatch(es)
2. Calibrated scale
3. Flat, measured walking surface with no sharp turns where the test performer will complete 1 mile (1.6 kilometers)
4. One heart rate monitor per test performer (if available)

Additional Personnel Needed: One or two test assistants

Setup:

1. The test performer is weighed (BW) without shoes and with minimal clothing (in kilograms).
2. The test performer is given a heart rate monitor. If a heart rate monitor is not available, the test performer will be paired with a test assistant or test partner.
3. The test administrator explains to the test performer the benefits of maintaining a constant pace and not starting too fast. The test performer should understand that he or she should not walk in a group during this test. Each test performer is expected to give his or her best effort.
4. The test administrator explains to the test performer what constitutes the designated course.
5. If multiple test performers are being evaluated simultaneously, multiple test assistants may be necessary to assist the test administrator in determining the place each test performer finishes and the corresponding time.
6. The test performer may practice walking for speed before beginning this test. A

walk is where one foot is *constantly* in contact with the ground.

7. The test performer lines up behind the starting line.

Administration and Directions:

1. On the test administrator's "go" command, the test performer walks the designated course as fast as possible.
2. One trial is performed.

Scoring:

1. The test administrator documents the time in which the test performer finishes the course in minutes and seconds.
2. As the test performer completes the course, the test administrator obtains his or her heart rate. This is done by either the test administrator viewing the heart rate monitor *or* a test assistant obtaining the test performer's pulse for 15 seconds after finishing the course and multiplying that number by 4.
3. The heart rate obtained is put into the following formula to determine the

VO_{2max}. (Gender: male = 1; female = 0. Time in minutes and seconds: seconds are divided by 60. For example, 13 minutes and 40 seconds is converted to 13.66.)

$$VO_{2max} = 132.853 - 0.1692(\text{body mass in kg}) - 0.3877(\text{age in years}) + 6.315(\text{gender}) - 3.2649(\text{time in minutes}) - 0.1565(HR)$$

5. The VO_{2max} calculation is recorded as the final score.

Checklist: The test performer must

1. Not run
2. Not short-cut the course
3. Not walk in a group

References

Meredith, M. D., & Welk, C. J. *FITNESSGRAM®/ ACTIVITYGRAM® test administration manual* (4th ed.). Champaign, IL: Human Kinetics.

■ ROCKPORT 1-MILE (1.6-KILOMETER) FITNESS WALKING TEST

Objective: Estimate cardiorespiratory fitness

Age Range: Child to adult

Equipment Needed:

1. Stopwatch
2. Calibrated scale
3. Heart rate monitor
4. One-mile-long flat, measured walking surface with no sharp turns

Additional Personnel Needed: One or two test assistants

Setup:

1. The test administrator explains to the test performer the benefits of maintaining a constant pace and not starting too fast. Multiple test performers should not walk in groups during this test. Each test performer is expected to give his or her best effort.
2. The test performer is given a heart rate monitor.

3. If a heart rate monitor is not available, the test performer should practice obtaining his or her pulse at the carotid artery before the test is administered.
4. The test performer may practice walking for speed before beginning this test. A walk is where one foot is *constantly* in contact with the ground.
5. The test performer lines up behind the starting line.

Administration and Directions:

1. On the test administrator's "go" command, the test performer walks the designated course as fast as possible at a steady pace.
2. One trial is performed.

Scoring:

1. If a heart rate monitor is utilized, the test administrator documents the test performer's heart rate when he or she crosses the finish line.
2. If a heart rate monitor is not utilized, a test assistant has the test performer measure his or her carotid pulse for 10 seconds, then multiplies that number by 6. This procedure results in scores that are not as accurate as those obtained by a heart rate monitor; the test performer's VO_{2max} may be overestimated.
3. The test performer's final walk time is recorded.
4. Heart rate, body mass, and time are put into the following formula to determine the VO_{2max}. (Gender: male = 1; female = 0. Time in minutes and seconds: seconds are divided by 60. For example, 13 minutes and 40 seconds is converted to 13.66.)

$$VO_{2max} = 132.853 - 0.1692(\text{body mass in kg}) - 0.3877(\text{age in years}) + 6.315(\text{gender}) - 3.2649(\text{time in minutes}) - 0.1565(HR)$$

5. The VO_{2max} calculation is recorded as the final score.

Checklist: The test performer must

1. Not run
2. Not short-cut the course
3. Not walk in a group

References

American College of Sports Medicine (2003). *ACSM's fitness book* (3rd ed.) Champaign, IL: Human Kinetics.

American College of Sports Medicine. (2006). *ACSM's guidelines for exercise testing and prescription* (7th ed.). Philadelphia: Lippincott Williams & Wilkins.

Dolgener, F. A., Hensley, L. D., Marsh, J. J., & Fjelstul, J. K. (1994). Validation of the Rockport fitness walking test in college males and females. *Research Quarterly for Exercise and Sport, 65*(2), 152–158.

Drowatzky, K. L., & Anders, F. F. (1996). Comparison of the Rockport walking and Cooper walk-run fitness tests. *Clinical Kinesiology, 50*(2), 36–39.

Heyward, V. H. (2006). *Advanced fitness assessment and exercise prescription* (5th ed.). Champaign, IL: Human Kinetics.

Kittredge, J. M., Rimmer, J. H., & Looney, M. A. (1994). Validation of the Rockport fitness walking test for adults with mental retardation. *Medicine and Science in Sports and Exercise, 26*(1), 95–102.

Kline, G. M., Porcari, J. P., Hintermeister, R., Freedson, P. S., Ward, A., McCarron, R. F., Ross, J., & Prentice, W. E. (1997). *Fitness for college and life* (5th ed.). St. Louis: Mosby.

Rippe, J. M. (1987). Estimation of VO_{2max} from a one-mile walk, gender, age, and body weight. *Medicine and Science in Sports and Exercise, 19*(3), 253–259.

Rippe, J. M., Ward, A., & Dougherty, K. (1986) *The Rockport Walking Program*. New York: Prentice Hall.

■ 3-MILE (4.8-KILOMETER) WALK TEST

Objective: Measure cardiorespiratory fitness

Age Range: 13 to 60+ (typically given to individuals who are unable or unfit to perform a running test)

Equipment Needed:

1. Stopwatch
2. Flat, measured walking surface with no sharp turns where the test performer can complete 3 miles (4.8 kilometers)

Additional Personnel Needed: One or two test assistants

Setup:

1. The test administrator explains to the test performer the benefits of maintaining a constant pace and not starting too fast. Multiple test performers should not walk in a group during this test. Each test performer is expected to give his or her best effort.
2. If multiple test performers are being evaluated simultaneously, multiple test assistants may be necessary to assist the test administrator in determining the place each test performer finishes and the corresponding time.
3. The test performer may need to practice walking for speed before beginning

this test. A walk is where one foot is *constantly* in contact with the ground.

4. The test performer lines up behind the starting line.

Administration and Directions:

1. On the test administrator's "go" command, the test performer walks the designated course as fast as possible.
2. One trial is performed.

Scoring:

1. The test administrator documents the time in which the test performer finishes the course in minutes and seconds.
2. The time is recorded as the final score.

Checklist: The test performer must

1. Not run
2. Not short-cut the course
3. Not walk in a group

Reference

Miller, D. K. (2006). *Measurement by the physical educator: Why and how* (5th ed.). New York: McGraw-Hill.

■ 6-MINUTE WALK TEST

Objective: Measure cardiorespiratory fitness

Age Range: Child to 60+ (designed for seniors, but may be given to other individuals who are unable or unfit to perform a running test)

Equipment Needed:

1. Stopwatch

2. Flat, open walking area (e.g., gym floor, hallway, room), with no sharp turns that can be observed by the test administrator
3. Four cones (or similar markers)
4. Tape
5. Chairs

6. Tape measure
7. Multiple tongue depressors (or similar light objects)

Additional Personnel Needed: One or two test assistants

Setup:

1. A 50-yard (45.7-meter) rectangular course is created with one cone placed in each corner and a strip of tape every 5 yards (4.5 meters) from the starting line. It should be easy for the test administrator to determine the distance the test performer travels (**Figure 8-1**).
2. Several chairs should be placed around the course.
3. The test administrator explains to the test performer the benefits of maintaining a constant pace and not starting too fast. Multiple test performers should not walk in a group during this test. Each test performer is expected to give his or her best effort.
4. If multiple test performers are being evaluated simultaneously, multiple test assistants may be necessary to assist the test administrator in determining the number of laps each test performer completes and the final distance traveled.
5. Test performers may need to practice walking for speed before beginning this test. A walk is where one foot is *constantly* in contact with the ground.
6. The test performer lines up behind the starting line.

Administration and Directions:

1. On the test administrator's "go" command, the test performer walks the designated course as fast as possible (refer to Figure 8-1).
2. A test performer who needs to rest during the test may utilize a chair until he or she feels comfortable continuing the test.

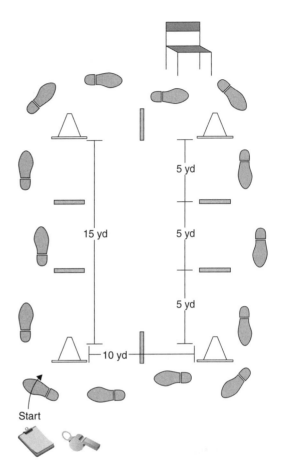

Figure 8-1   6-Minute Walk Test Setup and Administration

3. As a test performer passes the starting line, a test assistant should either give him or her tongue depressor or otherwise document that a lap was completed.
4. If multiple test performers are tested, a staggered start (one test performer beginning the test every 10 seconds) may be necessary.
5. The test performer continues walking for 6 minutes.

6. When the test administrator gives the "stop" command, the test performer stops and remains where he or she is until the position can be properly documented by the test administrator or a test assistant.
7. One trial is performed.

Scoring:

1. The test administrator adds the total distance walked by the test performer in 6 minutes to the nearest 5 yards (4.5 meters).
2. Each lap completed is equivalent to 50 yards (45.7 meters). The final lap is documented and added to the lap total.
3. Test performers who complete less than 328 yards (300 meters) during this test demonstrate poor cardiovascular capacity/fitness.
4. The total distance traveled is recorded as the final score.

Checklist: The test performer must

1. Not run
2. Not short-cut the course
3. Not walk in a group

References

American College of Sports Medicine. (2006). *ACSM's guidelines for exercise testing and prescription* (7th ed.). Philadelphia: Lippincott Williams & Wilkins.

ATS statement: Guidelines for the six-minute walk test. (2002). *American Journal of Respiratory Critical Care Medicine, 166,* 111–117.

Bitter, V., Weiner, D. H., Yusuf, S., Rogers, W. J., et al. (1993). Prediction of mortality and morbidity with a 6-minute walk test in patients with left ventricular dysfunction. *JAMA, 270*(14), 1702–1707.

Calders, P., Deforche, B., Verschelde, S., Bouckaert, J., et al. (2008). Predictors of 6-minute walk test and 12-minute walk/run test in obese children and adolescents. *European Journal of Pediatrics, 167,* 563–568.

Cavani, V., Mier, C. M., Musto, A. A., & Tummers, N. (2002). Effects of a 6-week resistance-training program on functional fitness of older adults. *Journal of Aging and Physical Activity, 10,* 443–452.

Enright, P. L. (2003). The six-minute walk test. *Respiratory Care, 48*(8), 783–785.

Guyatt, G. H., Sullivan, M. J., Thompson, P. J., et al. (1985). The 6-minute walk: A new measure of exercise capacity in patients with chronic heart failure. *Canadian Medical Association Journal, 132,* 919–923.

Jurimae, T., Rehand, M., Jurimae, J., Pihl, E., Gross, A., & Tammik, K. (2001). An influence of physical activity level and anthropometric indices on the 6-minute walking test results in elderly females. *Biology of Sport, 18*(2), 137–145.

Morrow, J. R., Jackson, A. W., Disch, J. G., & Mood, D. P. (2005). *Measurement and evaluation in human performance* (3rd ed.). Champaign, IL: Human Kinetics.

Rikli, R. E., & Jones, C. J. (1999). Development and validation of a functional fitness test for community-residing older adults. *Journal of Aging and Physical Activity, 7,* 129–161.

Rikli, R. E., & Jones, C. J. (1999). Functional fitness normative scores for community-residing older adults, ages 60–94. *Journal of Aging and Physical Activity, 7,* 162–182.

Rikli, R. E., & Jones, C. J. (2001). *Senior fitness test manual.* Champaign, IL: Human Kinetics.

■ 2-MINUTE STEP-IN-PLACE TEST

Objective: Measure cardiorespiratory fitness in an elderly population

Age Range: 60 to 90+ (generally performed for individuals who cannot, or would not, complete the 6-minute walk test)

Equipment Needed:

1. Stopwatch
2. Tape measure
3. Tape
4. Wall

Additional Personnel Needed: Test assistant

Setup:

1. The test performer stands with the *right* side closest to the wall.
2. The height of the test performer's patella midpoint and the iliac crest is measured and marked on the wall with tape.
3. The distance between the marks is measured and divided by 2. This result is marked on the wall approximately 2 feet forward of the original two marks.
4. This third mark represents the knee-step height specific to this test performer. It should be level with the midpoint between the middle of the patella and the iliac crest.
5. This knee-step height may be marked by other means (e.g., ruler taped to a chair, books, adjustable stand).
6. The test performer may practice the step height and pattern (described below) for one to three complete steps to become accustomed to the motion and height.

Administration and Directions:

1. On the test administrator's "go" command, the test performer begins stepping in place one leg at a time, starting with the *right* leg and alternating to the left leg. The patella should be brought to the height of the knee-step height determined earlier (**Figure 8-2**).
2. The test performer steps continuously for 2 minutes.
3. One trial is performed.

Scoring:

1. Although the test performer steps with both legs, only the *right* leg is used in scoring.
2. The number of proper steps to the measured knee-step height completed by the *right* leg in 2 minutes is counted and recorded. This number is recorded as the final score.

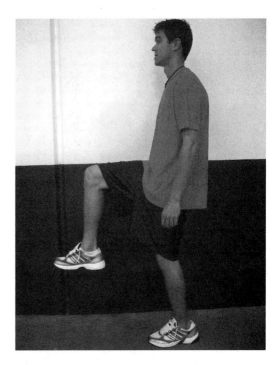

Figure 8-2 2-Minute Step-in-Place Test Administration

Checklist: The test performer must

1. Understand this is an endurance test and should not start too fast
2. Have good one-leg balance before this test is conducted

References

Morrow, J. R., Jackson, A. W., Disch, J. G., & Mood, D. P. (2005). *Measurement and evaluation in human performance* (3rd ed.). Champaign, IL: Human Kinetics.

Rikli, R. E., & Jones, C. J. (1999). Development and validation of a functional fitness test for community-residing older adults. *Journal of Aging and Physical Activity, 7,* 129–161.

Rikli, R. E., & Jones, C. J. (1999). Functional fitness normative scores for community-residing older adults, ages 60–94. *Journal of Aging and Physical Activity, 7,* 162–182.

Rikli, R. E., & Jones, C. J. (2001). *Senior fitness test manual.* Champaign, IL: Human Kinetics.

■ YMCA 3-MINUTE STEP TEST

Objective: Measure cardiovascular fitness with a submaximal step test

Age Range: 18 to 60+

Equipment Needed:

1. Stopwatch
2. Metronome
3. Stable bench or platform 12 inches (30.5 centimeters) high

Additional Personnel Needed: One test assistant or test partner per test performer

Setup:

1. Each test performer is paired with another test performer or a test assistant.
2. The test performers practice obtaining each other's pulse at the carotid artery before the test is administered.
3. The metronome is set to 96 beats per minute (24 steps per minute).
4. The test performer is allowed to practice the proper step pattern (described below) for 15 to 20 seconds to become accustomed to the motion, pace, and stepping with the metronome.
5. The test performer then stops practicing and lines up on the ground facing the bleachers. The bleachers should be within stepping distance.

Administration and Directions:

1. On the test administrator's "go" command, the test performer begins moving in step with the metronome.
2. The proper step pattern is "up" (right foot), "up" (left foot), "down" (left foot), "down" (right foot). Each time the test performer steps up onto and down off of the bleacher, the knee must be fully extended. To avoid excessive fatigue on the lead leg, it is permissible to occasionally change the lead leg during the test.
3. The test performer steps continuously for 3 minutes.

4. At the conclusion of the test, the test performer quickly sits down while the test partner or assistant obtains the test performer's carotid pulse. The test performer remains seated for the duration of the pulse attainment process.
5. One trial is performed.

Scoring:

1. The test partner or assistant obtains the test performer's carotid pulse for 1 minute.
2. The carotid pulse is recorded as the final score.

Checklist: The test performer must

1. Stay in step with the cadence (if multiple test performers are tested simultaneously, they all should step together)

2. Bring the body fully onto and off of the bleachers with each complete step
3. Sit immediately after the trial and remain seated until the pulse is taken

References

American College of Sports Medicine. (2006). *ACSM's guidelines for exercise testing and prescription* (7th ed.). Philadelphia: Lippincott Williams & Wilkins.

Golding, L. A. (2000). *YMCA fitness testing and assessment manual* (4th ed.). Champaign, IL: Human Kinetics.

Miller, D. K. (2006). *Measurement by the physical educator: Why and how* (5th ed.). New York: McGraw-Hill.

■ QUEENS COLLEGE STEP TEST

Objective: Measure cardiorespiratory fitness by performing a submaximal step test

Age Range: College age

Equipment Needed:

1. Stopwatch
2. Metronome
3. Gymnasium bleachers or a flight of stairs 16.25 inches (42.2 cm) high

Additional Personnel Needed: One test assistant or test partner per test performer

Setup:

1. Males and females are separated into two groups, as each has a different cadence.
2. Each test performer is paired with another test performer or a test assistant.

A male paired with a female is preferable because they will be tested separately.

3. The test performers practice obtaining each other's pulses at the carotid artery before the test is administered.
4. The metronome is set to the proper cadence.

   Males: 96 beats per minute (24 steps per minute)

   Females: 88 beats per minute (22 steps per minute)

5. The test performer is allowed to practice the proper step pattern (described below) for 15 to 20 seconds to become accustomed to the motion, pace, and stepping with the metronome.

6. The test performer then stops practicing and lines up on the ground facing the bleachers. The bleachers should be within stepping distance.

Administration and Directions:

1. On the test administrator's "go" command, the test performer begins moving in step with the metronome.
2. The proper step pattern is "up" (right foot), "up" (left foot), "down" (left foot), "down" (right foot). Each time the test performer steps up onto and down off of the bleacher, the knee must be fully extended. To avoid excessive fatigue on the lead leg, it is permissible to occasionally change the lead leg during the test.
3. The test performer steps continuously for 3 minutes.
4. At the conclusion of the test, the test performer remains standing while the test partner finds the test performer's carotid pulse (this should take no more than 5 seconds).
5. One trial is performed.

Scoring:

1. Once the test partner finds the test performer's carotid pulse, the test administrator tells the test partner to start counting the carotid pulse for 15 seconds. For best results, the test performer's pulse should be measured within 20 seconds after the test performer concludes the trial.
2. The 15-second carotid pulse is multiplied by 4; this is the recovery heart rate (RHR).
3. The pulse is recorded as the final score.
4. This score may be converted to a VO_{2max} and recorded as the final score.

> Men: $VO_{2max} = 111.33 - (0.42 \times RHR)$

> Women: $VO_{2max} = 65.81 - (0.1847 \times RHR)$

Checklist: The test performer must

1. Stay in step with the specific cadence (if multiple test performers are tested simultaneously, they all should step together)
2. Bring the body fully onto and off of the bleachers with each complete step
3. Remain standing after the trial so that the test partner may obtain the carotid pulse

References

Ashley, C. D., Smith, J. F., & Reneau, P. D. (1997). A modified step test based on a function of subjects' stature. *Perceptual and Motor Skills, 85,* 987–993.

Bandyopadhyay, A. (2007). Queen's College step test: An alternative of Harvard step test in young Indian men. *International Journal of Applied Sports Sciences, 19*(2), 1–6.

Chatterjee, S., Chatterjee, P., Mukherjee, P. S., & Bandyopadhyay, A. (2004). Validity of Queen's College step test for use with young Indian men. *British Journal of Sports Medicine, 38,* 289–291.

Johnson, B. L., & Nelson, J. K. (1986). *Practical measurements for evaluation in physical education* (4th ed.). New York: MacMillan.

Katch, F. L., & McArdle, W. D. (1983). *Nutrition, weight control, and exercise* (2nd ed.). Philadelphia: Lea & Febiger.

McArdle, W. D., Katch, F. I., Pechar, G. S., Jacobson, L., & Ruck, S. (1972). Reliability and interrelationships between maximal oxygen intake, physical work capacity, and step test scores in college women. *Medicine and Sciences in Sports, 4*(4), 182–186.

Miller, D. K. (2006). *Measurement by the physical educator: Why and how* (5th ed.). New York: McGraw-Hill.

Tritschler, K. (2000). *Barrow & McGee's practical measurement and assessment* (5th ed.). Philadelphia: Lippincott Williams & Wilkins.

■ HARVARD STEP TEST

Objective: Measure cardiorespiratory fitness by estimating the capacity of the body to adjust to and recover from hard work

Age Range: College age (performed with males)

Equipment Needed:

1. Stopwatch
2. Metronome
3. Stable bench or platform 20 inches (50.8 centimeters) high

Additional Personnel Needed: One test assistant or test partner per test performer

Setup:

1. Each test performer is paired with another test performer or a test assistant.
2. If test partners are used, they should practice obtaining each other's pulses at the carotid artery before the test is administered.
3. The metronome is set to 120 beats per minute (30 steps per minute).
4. The test performer is allowed to practice the proper step pattern (described below) for 15 to 20 seconds to become accustomed to the motion, pace, and stepping with the metronome.
5. The test performer then stops practicing and lines up on the ground facing the bleachers. The bleachers should be within stepping distance.

Administration and Directions:

1. On the test administrator's "go" command, the test performer begins moving in step with the metronome.
2. The proper step pattern is "up" (right foot), "up" (left foot), "down" (left foot), "down" (right foot). Each time the test

performer steps up onto and down off of the bleacher, the knee must be fully extended. To avoid excessive fatigue on the lead leg, it is permissible to occasionally change the lead leg during the test.
3. The test performer steps continuously for 5 minutes.
4. At the conclusion of the test, the test performer quickly sits down while the test partner or assistant obtains the test performer's carotid pulse. The test performer remains seated for the duration of the pulse attainment process.
5. One trial is performed.

Scoring: This test can be scored in two forms to calculate the physical efficiency index (PEI): long form or short form.

1. Long form: Pulse is obtained for 30 seconds on three occasions after exercise and utilized to calculate the PEI as described below.

   1 minute after exercise (1 to 1.5 minutes)
   2 minutes after exercise (2 to 2.5 minutes)
   3 minutes after exercise (3 to 3.5 minutes)

   PEI = (duration of exercise in seconds × 100) ÷ (2 × sum of pulse counts in recovery)

   PEI standards for long form:

   <55 = poor
   55 to 64 = low-average
   65 to 79 = high-average
   80 to 89 = good
   >89 = excellent

2. Short form: One minute to 1.5 minutes after exercise, the pulse is obtained for

30 seconds and used to calculate the PEI as described below.

> PEI =   (duration of exercise in seconds
>   × 100) ÷ (5.5 × pulse count from
>   1 to 1.5 minutes after exercise)

PEI standards for short form:

<50 = poor
50 to 80 = average
>80 = good

3. If a test performer does not complete the 5-minute test, the scoring below may be used to correspond to the individual's PEI.

<2 minutes = 25
2 to 3 minutes = 38
3 to 3.5 minutes = 48
3.5 to 4 minutes = 52
4 to 4.5 minutes = 55
4.5 to 5 minutes = 59

4. The PEI is recorded as the final score.

Checklist: The test performer must

1. Stay in step with the cadence (if multiple test performers are tested simultaneously, they all should step together)

2. Bring the body fully onto and off of the bleachers with each complete step

3. Sit immediately after the trial and remain seated until the pulse is taken

References

Brodie, D. A. (1996). *A reference manual for human performance measurement in the field of physical education and sports sciences.* Lewiston, NY: Edwin Mellen Press.

Brouha, L. (1943). The step test: A simple method of measuring physical fitness for muscular work in young men. *Research Quarterly, 14,* 31–36.

Bucher, C. A., & Prentice, W. E. (1985). *Fitness for college and life.* St. Louis: Mosby.

Cooke, W. P., & Holt, L. E. (1974). The effects of weight and leg length on Harvard step-test performance, utilizing stepping heights of 17, 20, and 23 inches. *American Corrective Therapy Journal, 28*(5), 142–144.

Johnson, B. L., & Nelson, J. K. (1986). *Practical measurements for evaluation in physical education* (4th ed.). New York: MacMillan.

Miller, D. K. (2006). *Measurement by the physical educator: Why and how* (5th ed.). New York: McGraw-Hill.

■ HARVARD STEP TEST FOR JUNIOR AND SENIOR HIGH MALES

Objective: Measure cardiorespiratory fitness by estimating the capacity of the body to adjust to and recover from hard work

Age Range: Males 12 to 18 years

Equipment Needed:

1. Calibrated scale

2. Tape measure or similar apparatus to measure body height

3. Stopwatch

4. Metronome

5. Stable bench or platform 18 *or* 20 inches high (45.7 *or* 50.8 centimeters)

Additional Personnel Needed: One test assistant or test partner per test performer

Setup:

1. The test administrator measures the test performer's weight. The test performer should not be wearing shoes and should be wearing a minimum of clothing.

2. The test administrator measures the test performer's height. The test performer should not be wearing shoes and should be standing erect.

3. The test administrator uses a nonogram (**Figure 8-3**) to determine the test performer's total body surface area. The

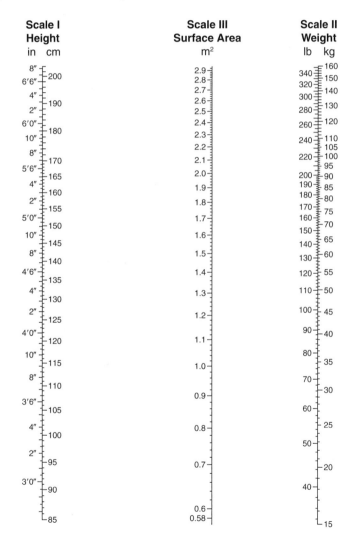

Figure 8-3 Total Body Surface Area Nonogram

Source: Reproduced from *Fitness for college and life*, Fifth edition. Prentice, W. E., pg. 225. Copyright Elsevier (1997).

test performer's total body surface area determines the test performer's test step height. To use the nomogram, place a ruler connecting the test performer's height and weight. The point where the ruler intersects the center column is the test performer's total surface area.

4. Test performers with a total body surface area less than 1.85 square meters utilize an 18-inch (45.7-cm) bench.
5. Test performers with a total body surface area greater than 1.85 square meters utilize a 20-inch (50.8-cm) bench.
6. Each test performer is paired with another.
7. The test partners practice obtaining each other's pulses at the carotid artery before the test is administered.
8. The metronome is set to the cadence of 120 beats per minute (30 steps per minute).
9. The test performer is allowed to practice the proper step pattern (described below) for 15 to 20 seconds to become accustomed to the motion, pace, and stepping with the metronome.
10. The test performer stops practicing and lines up on the ground facing the bleachers within stepping distance.

Administration and Directions:

1. On the test administrator's "go" command, the test performer begins moving in step with the metronome.
2. The proper step pattern is "up" (right foot), "up" (left foot), "down" (left foot), "down" (right foot). Each time the test performer steps up onto and down off of the bleacher, the knee must be fully extended. To avoid excessive fatigue on the lead leg, it is permissible to occasionally change the lead leg during the test.

3. The test performer steps continuously for 4 minutes.
4. At the conclusion of the test, the test performer quickly sits down so the test partner can obtain the test performer's carotid pulse. The test performer remains seated for the duration of the pulse attainment process.
5. One trial is performed.

Scoring:

1. The test performer's pulse is obtained for 30 seconds on three occasions after exercise: 1 minute after exercise (1 to 1.5 minutes), 2 minutes after exercise (2 to 2.5 minutes), and 3 minutes after exercise (3 to 3.5 minutes). The pulse is utilized to calculate the physical efficiency index (PEI) as described below.

$$\text{PEI} = \frac{\text{(duration of exercise in seconds} \times 100)}{(2 \times \text{sum of pulse counts in recovery)}}$$

PEI standards:

<55 = very poor
51 to 60 = poor
61 to 70 = fair
71 to 80 = good
81 to 90 = excellent
>92 = superior

2. The PEI is recorded as the final score.

Checklist: The test performer must

1. Stay in step with the specific cadence (if multiple test performers are tested simultaneously, they all should step together)
2. Bring the body fully onto and off of the bleachers with each complete step
3. Sit immediately after the trial and remains seated until the pulse is obtained

References

Gallagher, J. R., & Brouha, L. (1943). A simple method of testing the physical fitness of boys. *Research Quarterly, 14,* 23–30.

Miller, D. K. (2006). *Measurement by the physical educator: Why and how* (5th ed.). New York: McGraw-Hill.

Prentice, W. E. (1997). *Fitness for college and life* (5th ed.). St. Louis: Mosby.

■ HARVARD STEP TEST FOR JUNIOR HIGH, SENIOR HIGH, AND COLLEGE FEMALES

Objective: Measure cardiorespiratory fitness by estimating the capacity of the body to adjust to and recover from hard work

Age Range: Females 12 to 25 years

Equipment Needed:

1. Stopwatch
2. Metronome
3. Stable bench or platform 18 inches (45.7 centimeters) high

Additional Personnel Needed: One test assistant or test partner per test performer

Setup:

1. Each test performer is paired with another.
2. The test partners practice obtaining each other's pulses at the carotid artery before the test is administered.
3. The metronome is set to the cadence of 96 beats per minute (24 steps per minute).
4. The test performer is allowed to practice the step pattern (described below) for 15 to 20 seconds to become accustomed to the motion, pace, and stepping with the metronome.
5. The test performer stops practicing and lines up on the ground facing the bleachers within stepping distance.

Administration and Directions:

1. On the test administrator's "go" command, the test performer begins moving in step with the metronome.
2. The proper step pattern is "up" (right foot), "up" (left foot), "down" (left foot), "down" (right foot). Each time the test performer steps up onto and down off of the bleacher, the knee must be fully extended. To avoid excessive fatigue on the lead leg, it is permissible to occasionally change the lead leg during the test.
3. The test performer steps continuously for 3 minutes.
4. At the conclusion of the test, the test performer quickly sits down while the test partner obtains the test performer's carotid pulse. The test performer remains seated for the duration of the pulse attainment process.
5. One trial is performed.

Scoring: This test can be scored two ways: fitness index (FI) or cardiovascular efficiency score (CES).

1. FI: Pulse is obtained for 30 seconds on three occasions after exercise: 1 minute after exercise (1 to 1.5 minutes),

2 minutes after exercise (2 to 2.5 minutes), and 3 minutes after exercise (3 to 3.5 minutes). The pulse is utilized to calculate the FI:

> FI = (duration of exercise in seconds × 100) ÷ (2 × sum of pulse counts in recovery)

2. CES: One minute after exercise, the pulse is obtained for 30 seconds (recovery pulse). The pulse is utilized to calculate the CES as described below.

> CES = (duration of test in seconds × 100) ÷ (recovery pulse × 5.6)

3. The FI or CES is recorded as the final score.

Checklist: The test performer must

1. Stay in step with the specific cadence (if multiple test performers are tested simultaneously, they all should step together)

2. Bring the body fully onto and off of the bleachers on each complete step
3. Sit immediately after the trial and remain seated until the pulse is taken

References

Ganeriwal, S. K., Sen, S. C., & Khandare, S. S. (1968). Test of physical fitness (Harvard step test) in Indian females. *Indian Journal of Medical Research, 56*(6), 845–849.

Johnson, B. L., & Nelson, J. K. (1986). *Practical measurements for evaluation in physical education* (4th ed.). New York: MacMillan.

Miller, D. K. (2006). *Measurement by the physical educator: Why and how* (5th ed.). New York: McGraw-Hill.

Skubic, V., & Hodgkins, J. (1963). Cardiovascular efficiency test for girls and women. *Research Quarterly, 34,* 191–198.

Sloan, A. W. (1959). Modified Harvard step test for women. *Journal of Applied Physiology, 14*(6), 985–986.

■ HARVARD STEP TEST FOR ELEMENTARY SCHOOL-AGED MALES AND FEMALES

Objective: Measure cardiorespiratory by estimating the capacity of the body to adjust to and recover from hard work

Age Range: Elementary school age

Equipment Needed:

1. Stopwatch
2. Metronome
3. Stable bench or platform 14 inches (35.5 centimeters) high

Additional Personnel Needed: One test assistant or test partner per test performer

Setup:

1. The test administrator determines the age of each test performer.
2. Each test performer is paired with another test performer or a test assistant.
3. The test partners practice obtaining each other's pulses at the carotid artery before

the test is administered. Depending on the age of the test performers and their partners, an adult may be needed to accurately collect the pulse data.

4. The metronome is set to the cadence of 120 beats per minute (30 steps per minute).

5. The test performer is allowed to practice the proper step pattern (described below) for 15 to 20 seconds to become accustomed to the motion, pace, and stepping with the metronome.

6. The test performer stops practicing and lines up on the ground facing the bleachers within stepping distance.

Administration and Directions:

1. On the test administrator's "go" command, the test performer begins moving in step with the metronome.

2. The proper step pattern is "up" (right foot), "up" (left foot), "down" (left foot), "down" (right foot). Each time the test performer steps up onto and down off of the bleacher, the knee must be fully extended. To avoid excessive fatigue on the lead leg, it is permissible to occasionally change the lead leg during the test.

3. Test performers between 8 and 12 years old should step continuously for 3 minutes.

4. Test performers who are 7 years old should step continuously for 2 minutes.

5. At the conclusion of the test, the test performer quickly sits down so the test partner can obtain the test performer's carotid pulse. The test performer remains seated for the duration of the pulse attainment process.

6. One trial is performed.

Scoring: This test can be scored in two forms to calculate the physical efficiency index (PEI): long form or short form.

1. Long form: Pulse is obtained for 30 seconds on occasions after exercise: 1 minute after exercise (1 to 1.5 minutes), 2 minutes after exercise (2 to 2.5 minutes), and 3 minutes after exercise (3 to 3.5 minutes). The pulse is utilized to calculate the PEI as described below.

PEI = (duration of exercise in seconds × 100) ÷ (2 × sum of pulse counts in recovery)

PEI standards for long form:

<55 = poor
55 to 64 = low–average
65 to 79 = high–average
80 to 89 = good
>89 = excellent

2. Short form: One minute to 1.5 minutes after exercise, pulse is obtained for 30 seconds and used to calculate the PEI as described below.

PEI = (duration of exercise in seconds × 100) ÷ (5.5 × pulse count from 1 to 1.5 minutes after exercise)

PEI standards for short form:

<50 = poor
50 to 80 = average
>80 = good

3. If a test performer does not complete the 5-minute test, the scoring below may be used to correspond to the individual's PEI.

<2 minutes = 25
2 to 3 minutes = 38
3 to 3.5 minutes = 48
3.5 to 4 minutes = 52
4 to 4.5 minutes = 55
4.5 to 5 minutes = 59

4. The PEI is recorded as the final score.

Checklist: The test performer must

1. Stay in step with the specific cadence (if multiple test performers are tested simultaneously, they all should step together)
2. Bring the body fully onto and off of the bleachers with each complete step
3. Sit immediately after the trial and remain seated until the pulse is taken

References

Miller, D. K. (2006). *Measurement by the physical educator: Why and how* (5th ed.). New York: McGraw-Hill.

Tinsdall, F. F., Robertson, E. C., Drake, T. G. H., Jackson, S. H., et al. (1951). The Canadian Red Cross school meal study. *Canadian Medical Association Journal, 64*(6), 477–489.

■ HOOSIER ENDURANCE SHUTTLE RUN TEST

Objective: Measure cardiorespiratory fitness in children and teens

Age Range: 6 to 17

Equipment Needed:

1. Stopwatch
2. Tape measure
3. Two chairs (or similar objects)
4. Multiple (10 to 15) objects that can be easily grasped and run with (e.g., erasers, tape rolls)
5. Collection box
6. Flat, open running surface

Additional Personnel Needed: Test assistant

Setup:

1. The two chairs are placed 20 yards (18 meters) apart in a straight line.
2. The collection box is placed behind chair A.
3. A test assistant stands behind chair B with all of the objects.
4. The test performer stands behind chair A facing chair B (**Figure 8-4**).

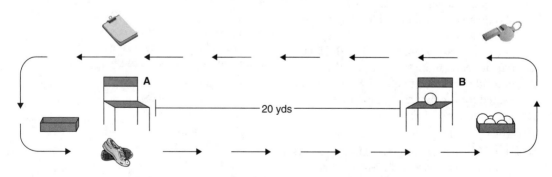

Figure 8-4   Hoosier Endurance Shuttle Run Test Setup and Administration

Administration and Directions:

1. On the test administrator's "go" command, the test performer runs from chair A to chair B and grasps the object that is placed on chair B (refer to Figure 8-4).
2. After the test performer grasps the object, he or she continues running *around* chair B and returns to *behind* chair A.
3. The test performer places the object into the collection box behind chair A.
4. The test performer continues running *around* chair A to chair B to grasp the next object.
5. Once the object is grasped off chair B, it is replaced by the test assistant.
6. This process continues for 6 minutes.
7. One trial is performed.

Scoring:

1. The number of objects successfully carried from chair B to the collection box is counted and recorded. Each object represents 40 yards (36.5 meters) traveled.

2. If the final object is grasped from chair B, but not placed in the collection box before time expires, that lap is counted as a complete lap.
3. If the final object is not grasped from chair B before time expires, the lap is not counted.
4. The total distance recorded as the final score.

Checklist: The test performer must

1. Understand this is an endurance test—test performers should pace themselves and not begin the test too fast
2. Go behind and around each chair
3. Place (not throw or toss) the object into the collection box

References

Miller, D. K. (2006). *Measurement by the physical educator: Why and how* (5th ed.). New York: McGraw-Hill.

Safrit, M. J. (1995). *Complete guide to youth fitness testing.* Champaign, IL: Human Kinetics.

■ PROGRESSIVE AEROBIC CARDIOVASCULAR ENDURANCE RUN (PACER) TEST

Objective: Measure aerobic capacity in a young population and teach children the concept of pacing

Age Range: Child

Equipment Needed:

1. Tape measure
2. Two cones
3. Open gym floor

4. CD containing the "beep" sequence (commercially available)
5. CD player

Additional Personnel Needed: Test assistant

Setup:

1. Since this test is performed with young children, the test administrator may need to conduct this test informally to

allow the test performers to understand fully how to perform this test. Practice will allow the test performers to better understand how to perform the test and what to expect from the test. The test administrator should return several days later to give the test and record the results.

2. Two cones are placed 20 meters (21.8 yards) apart in a straight line (**Figure 8-5**).

3. The CD player is placed on the course and the volume adjusted so that it can be heard easily on both lines during the test.

4. The test administrator explains to the test performer that this test begins slowly and gradually increases in difficulty.

5. The test performer lines up behind the first line. Multiple test performers, or an entire class, can be tested simultaneously.

6. The test administrator stands perpendicular to a line, and the test assistant stands perpendicular to the opposite line.

Administration and Directions:

1. The test administrator starts the CD.

2. The test performer listens to the CD and runs back and forth between the two lines every time a beep is heard. The pace of the beeps increases gradually during the test.

3. The test performer must touch the opposite line from where he or she started with the *foot* before the next beep is heard for the trial to be considered complete.

4. If the test performer reaches the opposite line before the next beep, he or she must remain at that side until the next beep is heard, prompting him or her to run to the opposite line.

5. If the test performer does not reach the opposite line before the next beep, the test performer reverses direction from where he or she is when the beep is heard and attempts to catch up with the test.

6. The test is stopped for the test performer when two total beeps are missed, whether the beeps are consecutive or not.

7. Because this test is typically performed with small children, the test administrator should ensure that the children who perform better on the test do not tease the children who do not.

8. The test performer, specifically at the beginning of the trial, does not need to sprint between cones.

9. One complete trial is performed.

Scoring:

1. Each completed 20-meter (21.8-yard) run is recorded as one lap.

2. The test administrator and test assistant document the lap number on which the test performer misses the second beep.

3. The number of laps successfully completed is recorded as the final score.

4. This figure can be converted into VO_{2max} and recorded as the final score by utilizing the following formula. (Max speed = 8.5 kilometers/hour (km/h) + 0.5 km/h for

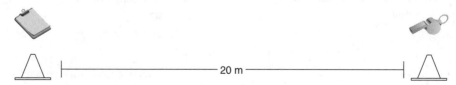

20 m

Figure 8-5 Progressive Aerobic Cardiovascular Endurance Run Test Setup

each stage successfully completed by the test performer.)

$$VO_{2max} = 31.025 + (3.238 \times \text{max speed}) - (3.248 \times \text{age}) + (0.1536 \times \text{max speed} \times \text{age})$$

Checklist: The test performer must

1. Not maximally sprint in the beginning of the test
2. Not run to the opposite line before the beep is heard
3. Walk and recover between beeps on the opposite line

There also is a 15-meter (16.4-yard) version of the PACER that can be utilized in smaller facilities.

References

Mahar, M. T., Rowe, D. S., Parker, C. P., Mahar, F. J., Dawson, M., & Holt, J. E. (1997). Criterion-referenced and norm-referenced agreement between the mile run/walk and PACER. *Measurement in Physical Education and Exercise Science, 1*(4), 245–258.

Mahar, M. T., Welk, G. J., Rowe, D. A., Crotts, D. J., & McIver, K. L. (2006). Development and validation of a regression model to estimate VO_{2max} from PACER 20-m shuttle run performance. *Journal of Physical Activity and Health, 3*(Suppl. 2), S34–S46.

McClain, J. J., Welk, G. J., Ihmels, M., & Schaben, J. (2006). Comparison of two versions of the PACER aerobic fitness test. *Journal of Physical Activity and Health,* 3(Suppl. 2), S47–S57.

Meredith, M. D., & Welk, C. J. *FITNESSGRAM®/ ACTIVITYGRAM® test administration manual* (4th ed.). Champaign, IL: Human Kinetics.

Safrit, M. J. (1995). *Complete guide to youth fitness testing.* Champaign, IL: Human Kinetics.

■ CONTINUOUS MULTISTAGE FITNESS (MFT) TEST

Also Known as: 20-Meter Shuttle Run (20-MSR) Test

Objective: Measure aerobic capacity

Age Range: High school to college age

Equipment Needed:

1. Tape measure
2. Two cones
3. Open field or gym floor
4. CD containing the beep sequence (commercially available)
5. CD player

Additional Personnel Needed: Test assistant

Setup:

1. Two cones are placed 20 meters (21.8 yards) apart in a straight line (**Figure 8-6**).
2. The CD player should be placed on the course and the volume adjusted so that it can be easily heard on both lines during the test.
3. The test administrator explains to the test performer that this test begins slowly and gradually increases in difficulty.

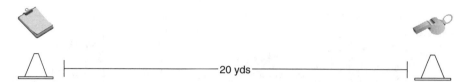

Figure 8-6 Continous Multistage Fitness Test Setup

4. The test performer lines up behind the first line. Multiple test performers, or an entire team, can be tested simultaneously.
5. The test administrator stands perpendicular to one line, while the test assistant stands perpendicular to the opposite line.

Administration and Directions:

1. The test administrator starts the CD.
2. The test performer listens to the CD and runs back and forth between the two lines every time a beep is heard. The pace is initially 8.5 kilometers per hour (kph) (5.28 miles per hour, mph) and increases by 0.5 kph (0.31 mph) every minute.
3. The test performer must reach the opposite line or be within 2 meters (2.2 yards) before the next beep occurs for the trial to be considered complete.
4. If the test performer reaches the opposite line before the next beep, he or she must remain at the line until the next beep is heard, prompting him or her to run to the opposite line.
5. If the test performer does not reach the opposite line before the next beep, he or she must continue running to the line, and then immediately turn and run to the opposite line, attempting to catch up with the test.
6. When the test performer misses two consecutive beeps, the test is stopped for the test performer.

7. The test performer, specifically at the beginning of the trial, does not need to sprint between cones.
8. One complete trial is performed.

Scoring:

1. A different level corresponds to every minute of the test. The test administrator knows the test performers have moved to a different level of the test because there will be an audible cue given on the CD.
2. The test administrator and test assistant document the level number and the shuttle number when the test performer fails to reach the opposite line two consecutive times.
3. The number of shuttles successfully completed on a specific level is recorded as the final score. For example, a score of 12 + 5 corresponds to the score for a test performer who completed five shuttles of level 12.
4. This figure can be converted into VO_{2max} and recorded as the final score by the following formula. (Max speed = 8.5 kph + 0.5 kph for each stage successfully completed by the test performer.)

$$VO_{2max} = 31.025 + (3.238 \times \text{max speed}) - (3.248 \times \text{age}) + (0.1536 \times \text{max speed} \times \text{age})$$

Checklist: The test performer must

1. Have an adequate level of conditioning before this test is performed

2. Not maximally sprint in the beginning of the test
3. Not run to the opposite line before the beep is heard
4. Walk and recover between beeps on the opposite line

References

Aziz, A. R., Mukherjee, S., Chia, M. Y. H., & Teh, K. C. (2008). Validity of the running repeated sprint ability test among playing positions and level of competitiveness in trained soccer players. *International Journal of Sports Medicine, 29*, 833–838.

Aziz, A. R., Yau, F. T. H., & Chuan, T. K. (2005). The 20m multistage shuttle run test: Reliability, sensitivity and its performance correlated in trained soccer players. *Asian Journal of Exercise and Sports Science, 2*(1), 1–7.

Berthoin, S., Gerbeaux, M., Turpin, E., Guerrin, F., Lensel-Corbeil, G., & Vandendorpe, F. (1994). Comparison of two field tests to estimate maximum aerobic speed. *Journal of Sports Sciences, 12*(4), 355–362.

Boreham, C. A. G., Paliczka, V. J., & Nichols, A. K. (1990). A comparison of the PWC170 and 20-MST test of aerobic fitness in adolescent schoolchildren. *Journal of Sports Medicine and Physical Fitness, 30*(1), 19–23.

Brodie, D. A. (1996). *A reference manual for human performance measurement in the field of physical education and sports sciences.* Lewiston, NY: Edwin Mellen Press.

Ekblom, B. (1994). *Football (soccer).* London: Blackwell Scientific Publications.

Gore, C. J. (2000). *Physiological tests for elite athletes.* Australian Sports Commission. Champaign, IL: Human Kinetics.

Leger, L. A., & Lambert, J. (1982). A maximal multistage 20-m shuttle run test to predict VO_{2max}. *European Journal of Applied Physiology, 49*, 1–12.

Leger, L. A., Mercier, D., Gadoury, C., & Lambert, J. (1988). The multistage 20 metre shuttle run test for aerobic fitness. *Journal of Sports Sciences, 6*, 93–101.

Ramsbottom, R., Brewer, J., & Williams, C. (1988). A progressive shuttle run test to estimate maximal oxygen uptake. *British Journal of Sports Medicine, 22*(4), 141–144.

St. Clair Gibson, A., Broomhead, S., Lambert, M. I., & Hawley, J. A. (1998). Prediction of maximal oxygen uptake from a 20-m shuttle run as measured directly in runners and squash players. *Journal of Sports Sciences, 16*, 331–335.

Svensson, M., & Drust, B. (2005). Testing soccer players. *Journal of Sports Sciences, 23*(6), 601–618.

Thomas, A., Dawson, B., & Goodman, C. (2006). The yo-yo test: Reliability and association with a 20-m shuttle run and VO_{2max}. *International Journal of Sports Physiology and Performance, 1*, 137–149.

■ YO-YO ENDURANCE (CONTINUOUS) TEST

Objective: Measure aerobic capacity and the ability to work continuously for a long period of time

Age Range: High school to college age

Equipment Needed:

1. Tape measure
2. Two cones
3. Open field or gym floor
4. CD containing the "beep" sequence (commercially available)
5. CD player

Additional Personnel Needed: Test assistant

Setup

1. The test administrator determines which level will be utilized.

   Level 1: Used for non-elite participants. The pace starts slower and increases gradually.

   Level 2: Used for elite participants. The pace starts faster and increases quicker than in level 1.

2. Two cones are placed 20 meters (21.8 yards) apart in a straight line (**Figure 8-7**).

3. The CD player should be placed on the course and the volume adjusted so that it can be easily heard on both lines during the test.

4. The test performer lines up behind the first line. Multiple test performers, or an entire team, can be tested simultaneously.

5. The test administrator stands perpendicular to the starting line, while the test assistant stands perpendicular to the opposite line.

Administration and Directions:

1. The test administrator starts the CD.

2. The test performer listens to the CD and runs back and forth between the two lines after a beep is heard. The pace of the beeps increases each minute.

3. The test performer must reach or be within 2 meters (2.2 yards) of the opposite line before the next beep occurs for the trial to be considered complete.

4. If the test performer reaches the opposite line before the next beep, he or she must remain at that side until the next beep is heard, prompting him or her to run to the other line.

5. If the test performer does not reach the opposite line before the next beep, he or she must continue running to the line, and then immediately turn and run to the opposite line, attempting to catch up with the test.

6. When the test performer misses two consecutive beeps, the test is stopped for the test performer.

7. The test performer, especially at the beginning of the trial, does not need to sprint between the cones.

8. One complete trial is performed.

Scoring:

1. The test administrator and test assistant document the level number and the shuttle number when the test performer fails to reach the opposite line two consecutive times.

2. The number of shuttles successfully completed on a specific level is recorded as the final score. For example, a score of 17 + 2 corresponds to the score for a test performer who completed 17 shuttles of level 2.

3. Alternatively, the total distance the test performer traversed can be recorded as the final score.

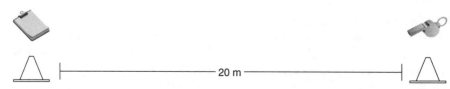

Figure 8-7   Yo-Yo Endurance Test Setup

Checklist: The test performer must

1. Have an adequate level of conditioning before this test is performed
2. Not maximally sprint in the beginning of the test
3. Not run to the opposite line before the beep is heard

References

Bangsbo, J. (1996). Yo-yo tests of practical endurance and recovery for soccer. *Performance Conditioning Soccer, 2*(9), 8.

Bangsbo, J., Mohr, M., Poulsen, A., Perez-Gomez, J., & Krustrup, P. (2006). Training and testing the elite athlete. *Journal of Exercise Science and Fitness, 4*(1), 1–14.

■ YO-YO INTERMITTENT ENDURANCE (YYIE) TEST

Objective: Measure aerobic capacity and ability to complete running intervals over a prolonged period of time; this test is useful for sports like tennis, basketball, and soccer

Age Range: High school to college age

Equipment Needed:

1. Tape measure
2. Three cones
3. Open field or gym floor
4. CD containing the "beep" sequence (commercially available)
5. CD player

Additional Personnel Needed: Test assistant

Setup:

1. The test administrator determines which level will be utilized.

   Level 1: Used for non-elite participants. The pace starts at 10 kilometers per hour (kph) (6.2 miles per hour [mph]) and increases gradually.

   Level 2: Used for elite participants. The pace starts at 13 kph (8 mph) and increases quicker than level 1.

2. Two cones are placed 20 meters (21.8 yards) apart in a straight line. The third cone (recovery cone) is placed 2.5 meters (2.7 yards) behind the starting cone (**Figure 8-8**).

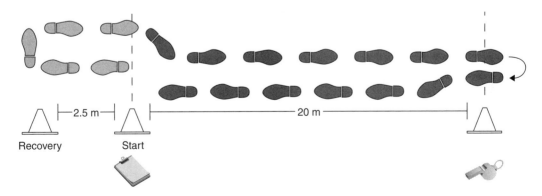

|←—2.5 m—→| |←————————— 20 m —————————→|

Recovery   Start

Figure 8-8 Yo-Yo Intermittent Endurance Test Setup

3. The CD player is placed on the course and the volume adjusted so that it can be easily heard on both lines during the test.
4. The test performer lines up behind the first line. Multiple test performers, or an entire team, can be tested simultaneously.
5. The test administrator stands perpendicular to the starting line, while the test assistant stands perpendicular to the opposite line.

Administration and Directions:

1. The test administrator starts the CD.
2. The test performer listens to the CD and runs back and forth between the two lines after a beep is heard. The pace of the beeps increases each minute.
3. The test performer must reach or be within 2 meters (2.2 yards) of the opposite line before the next beep occurs for the trial to be considered complete.
4. When the test performer returns to the starting line (after every two beeps), there is a 5-second rest period in which the test performer jogs around the recovery cone before the next series of two shuttles are run. This is cued on the CD.
5. If the test performer reaches the opposite line before the next beep, he or she must remain at that side until the next beep is heard, prompting him or her to run to the other line.
6. If the test performer does not reach the opposite line before the next beep, he or she must continue running to the line, then immediately turn and run to the opposite line, attempting to catch up with the test.
7. When the test performer misses two consecutive beeps, the test is stopped for the test performer.

8. The test performer, especially at the beginning of the trial, does not need to sprint between the cones.
9. One complete trial is performed.

Scoring:

1. The test administrator and test assistant document the level number and the shuttle number when the test performer fails to reach the opposite line two consecutive times.
2. The number of shuttles successfully completed on a specific level is recorded as the final score. For example, a score of 17 + 2 corresponds to the score for a test performer who completed 17 shuttles of level 2.
3. Alternatively, the total distance the test performer traversed can be recorded as the final score.

Checklist: The test performer must

1. Have an adequate level of conditioning before this test is performed
2. Not maximally sprint in the beginning of the test
3. Not run to the opposite line before the beep is heard
4. Walk and recover between beeps on the opposite line
5. Jog around the recovery cone after every two shuttles

References

Bangsbo, J. (1996). Yo-yo tests of practical endurance and recovery for soccer. *Performance Conditioning Soccer, 2*(9), 8.

Bangsbo, J. (2005). Learn more about the yo-yo intermittent endurance test. *Performance Conditioning Soccer, 11*(5), 7–8.

Bangsbo, J., Mohr, M., Poulsen, A., Perez-Gomez, J., & Krustrup, P. (2006). Training and testing the elite athlete. *Journal of Exercise Science and Fitness*, 4(1), 1–14.

Castagna, C., Impellizzeri, F. M., Belardinelli, R., et al. (2006). Cardiorespiratory responses to yo-yo intermittent endurance test in nonelite youth soccer players. *Journal of Strength and Conditioning Research*, 20(2), 326–330.

Castagna, C., Impellizzeri, F. M., Chamari, K., Carlomagno, D., & Rampinini, E. (2006). Aerobic fitness and yo-yo continuous and intermittent tests performances in soccer players: A correlation study. *Journal of Strength and Conditioning Research*, 20(2), 320–325.

Ekblom, B. (1994). *Football (soccer)*. London: Blackwell Scientific Publications.

Malina, R. M., Eisenmann, J. C., Cumming, S. P., Ribeiro, B., & Aroso, J. (2004). Maturity-associated variation in the growth and functional capacities of youth football (soccer) player 13–15 years. *European Journal of Applied Physiology*, 91, 555–562.

Metaxas, T. I., Koutlianos, N. A., Kouidi, E. J., & Deligiannis, A. P. (2005). Comparative study of field and laboratory tests for the evaluation of aerobic capacity in soccer players. *Journal of Strength and Conditioning Research*, 19(1), 79–84.

Svensson, M., & Drust, B. (2005). Testing soccer players. *Journal of Sports Sciences*, 23(6), 601–618.

■ YO-YO INTERMITTENT RECOVERY (YYIR) TEST

Objective: Measure aerobic capacity and ability to recover after intense exercise; this test is useful to assess fitness for activities that require the individual to perform intense exercise after short recovery periods, such as ice hockey, football, tennis, badminton, basketball, and soccer

Age Range: High school to college age

Equipment Needed:

1. Tape measure
2. Three cones
3. Open field or gym floor
4. CD containing the "beep" sequence (commercially available)
5. CD player

Additional Personnel Needed: Test assistant

Setup:

1. The test administrator determines which level will be utilized.

   Level 1: Used for non-elite participants. The pace starts at 10 kph (6.2 mph) and increases gradually.

   Level 2: Used for elite participants. The pace starts at 13 kph (8 mph) and increases quicker than in level 1.

2. Two cones are placed 20 meters (21.8 yards) apart in a straight line, the third cone (recovery cone) is placed 5 meters (5.4 yards) behind the starting cone (**Figure 8-9**).

3. The CD player should be placed on the course and the volume adjusted so that it can be easily heard on both lines during the test.

4. The test performer lines up behind the first line. Multiple test performers, or an entire team, can be tested simultaneously.

5. The test administrator stands perpendicular to the starting line, while the test assistant stands perpendicular to the opposite line.

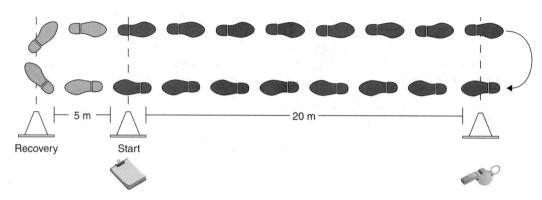

Figure 8-9 Yo-Yo Intermittent Recovery Test Setup

Administration and Directions:

1. The test administrator starts the CD.
2. The test performer listens to the CD and runs back and forth between the two lines after a beep is heard. The pace of the beeps increases each minute.
3. The test performer must reach or be within 2 meters (2.2 yards) of the opposite line before the next beep occurs for the trial to be considered complete.
4. When the test performer returns to the starting line (after every two beeps), there is a 10-second rest period in which the test performer jogs around the recovery cone before the next series of two shuttles is run. This is cued on the CD.
5. If the test performer reaches the opposite line before the next beep, he or she must remain at that side until the next beep is heard, prompting the performer to run to the other line.
6. If the test performer does not reach the opposite line before the next beep, he or she must continue running to the line, then immediately turn and run to the opposite line, attempting to catch up to the beep.

7. When the test performer misses two consecutive beeps, the test is stopped for the test performer.
8. The test performer, especially at the beginning of the trial, does not need to sprint between the cones.
9. One complete trial is performed.

Scoring:

1. The test administrator and test assistant document the level number and the shuttle number when the test performer fails to reach the opposite line two consecutive times.
2. The number of shuttles successfully completed on a specific level is recorded as the final score. For example, a score of 17 + 2 corresponds to the score for a test performer who completed 17 shuttles of level 2.
3. Alternatively, the total distance the test performer traversed can be recorded as the final score.
4. VO_{2max} can theoretically be estimated from the YYIR tests. Since the YYIR test does not exclusively test aerobic capacity

(partial anaerobic capacity), the formulas reported here are not considered extremely accurate.

YYIR Level 1: VO_{2max} = (distance in meters × 0.0084) + 36.4

YYIR Level 2: VO_{2max} = (distance in meters × 0.0136) + 45.3

Checklist: The test performer must

1. Have an adequate level of conditioning before this test is performed
2. Not maximally sprint in the beginning of the test
3. Not run to the opposite line before the beep is heard
4. Walk and recover between beeps on the opposite line
5. Jog around the recovery cone after every two shuttles

References

Atkins, S. J. (2006). Performance of the yo-yo intermittent recovery test by elite professional and semiprofessional rugby league players. *Journal of Strength and Conditioning Research, 20*(1), 222–225.

Bangsbo, J. (1996). Yo-yo tests of practical endurance and recovery for soccer. *Performance Conditioning Soccer, 2*(9), 8.

Bangsbo, J., Iaia, F. M., & Krustrup, P. (2008). The yo-yo intermittent recovery test: A useful tool for evaluation of physical performance in intermittent sports. *Sports Medicine, 38*(1), 37–51.

Bangsbo, J., Mohr, M., Poulsen, A., Perez-Gomez, J., & Krustrup, P. (2006). Training and testing the elite athlete. *Journal of Exercise Science and Fitness, 4*(1), 1–14.

Castagna, C., Abt, G., & D'Ottavio, S. (2005). Competitive-level differences in yo-yo intermittent recovery and twelve minute run test performance in soccer referees. *Journal of Strength and Conditioning Research, 19*(4), 805–809.

Castagna, C., Abt, G., & D'Ottavio, S. (2007). Physiological aspects of soccer refereeing performance and training. *Sports Medicine, 37*(1), 625–646.

Castagna, C., Impellizzeri, F. M., Chamari, K., Carlomagno, D., & Rampinini, E. (2006). Aerobic fitness and yo-yo continuous and intermittent tests performances in soccer players: A correlation study. *Journal of Strength and Conditioning Research, 20*(2), 320–325.

Krustrup, P., & Bangsbo, J. (2001). Physiological demands of top-class soccer refereeing in relation to physical capacity: Effect of intense intermittent exercise training. *Journal of Sports Sciences, 19*, 881–891.

Krustrup, P., Mohr, M., Amstrup, T., et al. (2003). The yo-yo intermittent recovery test: Physiological response, reliability, and validity. *Medicine and Science in Sports and Exercise, 35*, 697–705.

Metaxas, T. I., Koutlianos, N. A., Kouidi, E. J., & Deligiannis, A. P. (2005). Comparative study of field and laboratory tests for the evaluation of aerobic capacity in soccer players. *Journal of Strength and Conditioning Research, 19*(1), 79–84.

Mohr, M., Krustrup, P., & Bangsbo, J. (2003). Match performance of high-standard soccer players with special reference to development of fatigue. *Journal of Sports Sciences, 21*, 519–528.

Rostgaard, T., Iaia, F. M., Simonsen, D. S., & Bangsbo, J. (2008). A test to evaluate the physical impact on technical performance in soccer. *Journal of Strength and Conditioning Research, 22*(1), 283–292.

Sayers, A., Eveland Sayers, B., & Binkley, B. (2008). Preseason fitness testing in National Collegiate Athletic Association soccer. *Strength and Conditioning Journal, 30*(4), 70–75.

Stolen, T., Chamari, K., Castagna, C., & Wisloff, U. (2005). Physiology of soccer: An update. *Sports Medicine, 35*(6), 501–536.

Svensson, M., & Drust, B. (2005). Testing soccer players. *Journal of Sports Sciences, 23*(6), 601–618.

Thomas, A., Dawson, B., & Goodman, C. (2006). The yo-yo test: Reliability and association with a 20-m shuttle run and VO_{2max}. *International Journal of Sports Physiology and Performance, 1*, 137–149.

9

Anaerobic Capacity (Anaerobic Power) Testing

Anaerobic capacity, also termed anaerobic power, is the ability of the body to perform during and after intense exercises of moderate duration. Anaerobic capacity tests measure the ability of the test performer to clear lactic acid between trials and his or her ability to perform under conditions of increased lactic acid concentrations in the muscles. Anaerobic capacity tests involve continuous intense muscular activities lasting between 30 and 90 seconds with limited rest between test parts.

The test administrator should ensure the test performer properly warms up and stretches before an anaerobic capacity test. Anaerobic capacity tests require the test performer to engage in multiple trials of intense exercise with limited recovery time between test parts. The test performer should walk, stretch, and lightly jog between test parts while remaining alert to the announcement of the beginning of the subsequent test part(s). Doing so will help the test performer clear the lactic acid from the working muscles. At the conclusion of the anaerobic capacity test, the test performer should complete a proper cool-down session (i.e., through walking, light jogging, stretching). Anaerobic capacity tests are extremely fatiguing to perform and should be placed at the end of a test battery.

■ 60-YARD (54.8-METER) SHUTTLE TEST

Objective: Measure speed and anaerobic capacity

Age Range: High school to college age

Equipment Needed:

1. Stopwatch
2. Tape measure or lined American football field
3. Four cones
4. Flat, open surface at least 25 yards (22.8 meters) long; a lined American football field is ideal

Additional Personnel Needed: Test assistant

Setup:

1. Four cones are placed 5 yards (4.5 meters) apart in a straight line on the field (**Figure 9-1**).
2. The test performer is positioned behind one of the farthest cones (cone A).

3. A test assistant should be positioned on the course to ensure that the test performer completes the test properly.

Administration and Directions:

1. On the test administrator's "go" command, the test performer *sprints* to cone B, touching the line with the hand, then *sprints* to cone A, touching the line with the hand (refer to Figure 9-1).
2. Then the test performer turns and *sprints* to cone C, touching the line with the hand, then *sprints* back to cone A, touching the line with the hand.
3. The test performer next turns and *sprints* to cone D, touching the line with the hand, then *sprints* back past cone A.
4. Two trials may be performed.

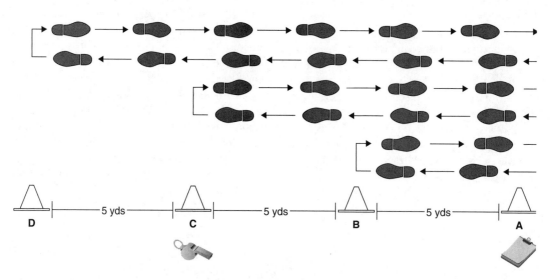

Figure 9-1   60-Yard Shuttle Test Setup and Administration

Scoring:

1. The shuttle times are recorded.
2. The best time is recorded as the final score.

Checklist: The test performer must

1. Maximally sprint during each shuttle
2. Touch the line at the end of each shuttle
3. Sprint through the finish line

References

Inside the Combine. (2008, February 20). *Chicago Tribune*, 5–7.

McGee, K. J., & Burkett, L. N. The National Football League Combine: A reliable predictor of draft status. *Journal of Strength and Conditioning Research, 17*(1), 6–11.

■ 300-YARD (274-METER) SHUTTLE TEST

Objective: Measure anaerobic capacity and recovery

Age Range: High school to college age

Equipment Needed:

1. Two stopwatches
2. Tape measure
3. Cones
4. Flat, open surface at least 25 yards (22.8 meters) long

Additional Personnel Needed: Two test assistants

Setup:

1. Two parallel lines are created 25 yards (22.8 meters) apart on a flat surface (**Figure 9-2**).
2. Test performers can be paired based on fitness levels if multiple individuals are being tested simultaneously.
3. The test performer is positioned behind the starting line.
4. A test assistant is positioned behind the opposite line.

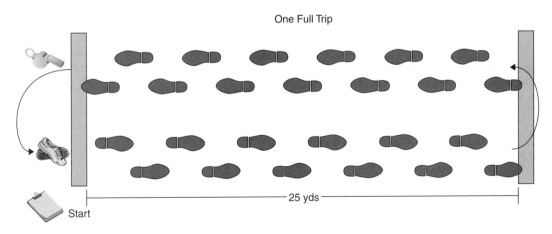

Figure 9-2   300-Yard Shuttle Test Setup and Administration

Administration and Directions

1. On the test administrator's "go" command, the test performer *sprints* to the opposite line, stops, and *sprints* back. Six complete trips are performed without rest (refer to Figure 9-2).
2. At the conclusion of the first shuttle (300 yards or 274 meters), the test performer's time is recorded and he or she is given 5 minutes to recover.
3. The test performer may walk, stretch, and consume fluids between trials but should remain alert for the start of the next shuttle.
4. After 5 minutes, the test performer begins the second shuttle in the same manner as the first.
5. One complete trial is performed.

Scoring:

1. Each shuttle time is recorded.
2. The closer the second shuttle is to the first shuttle, the better the test performer's anaerobic capacity.
3. The two times are averaged and recorded as the final score.

Checklist: The test performer must

1. Maximally sprint during each shuttle
2. Touch the line at the end of each shuttle
3. Actively recover between shuttles

References

Baechle, T. R., & Earle, R. W. (2008). *Essentials of strength training and conditioning* (3rd ed.). Champaign, IL: Human Kinetics.

Coaches roundtable: Testing for football. (1983). *National Strength and Conditioning Association Journal, 5*(5), 12–19.

Gilliam, G. M., & Marks, M. (1983). 300 yard shuttle run. *NSCA Journal, 5*(5), 46.

Jones, A. (1991). Test and measurement: 300-yard shuttle run. *National Strength and Conditioning Association Journal, 13*(2), 56.

Semenick, D. (1984). Anaerobic testing: Practical applications. *National Strength and Conditioning Association Journal, 6*(5), 45, 70–73.

Semenick, D., Connors, J., Carter, M., Harman, E., et al. (1992). Test and measurement: Rationale, protocols, testing/reporting forms and instructions for wrestling. *National Strength and Conditioning Association Journal, 14*(3), 54–59.

Sporis, G., Ruzic, L., & Leko, G. (2008). The anaerobic endurance of elite soccer players improved after a high-intensity training intervention in the 8-week conditioning program. *Journal of Strength and Conditioning Research, 22*(2), 559–566.

■ LINE DRILL TEST

Also Known as: Suicide Test/Drill

Objective: Measure anaerobic capacity and recovery

Age Range: High school to college age

Equipment Needed:

1. Two stopwatches
2. Standard (lined) basketball court

Additional Personnel Needed: One or two test assistants

Setup:

1. An entire standard basketball court is utilized for this test. Cones may be placed on the court for reference points. If a standard basketball court is not available, the test administrator can create a course with the same dimensions as a basketball court (**Figure 9-3**).

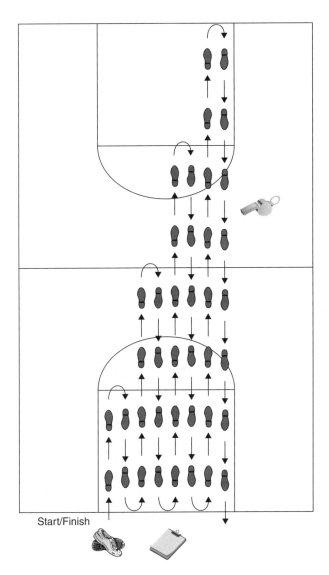

Start/Finish

Figure 9-3   Line Drill Test Setup and Administration

2. Test performers can be paired based on fitness levels if multiple individuals are being tested simultaneously.
3. A test assistant may be placed on the course to ensure the test performer executes the test protocol correctly.
4. The test performer begins behind the baseline designated the start/finish line.

Administration and Directions:

1. On the test administrator's "go" command, the test performer *sprints* to the nearest free-throw line, stops, and *sprints* back to the start/finish line (refer to Figure 9-3).
2. The test performer then stops and *sprints* to the half-court line, stops, and *sprints* back to the start/finish line.
3. The test performer then stops and *sprints* to the free-throw line farthest from the start/finish line, stops, and *sprints* back to the start/finish line.
4. The test performer then stops and *sprints* to the farthest baseline, stops, and *sprints* through the start/finish line.
5. A total of 452 feet (137.7 meters) is traversed during each line drill.
6. At the conclusion of the first line drill, the time is recorded, and the test performer is given 2 minutes to recover.
7. The test performer may walk, stretch, and consume fluids between line drills, but should remain alert for the start of the next line drill.
8. After the recovery period, the test performer begins the second line drill in the same manner as the first.
9. Four line drills are performed.
10. One complete trial is performed.

Scoring:

1. Each line drill time is recorded.
2. The closer the last trial is to the first, the better the test performer's anaerobic capacity.
3. The four times are averaged and recorded as the final score.

Checklist: The test performer must

1. Understand how to run the course
2. Touch each line with the foot before changing directions
3. Sprint straight during each trial
4. Actively recover between shuttles

References

Baechle, T. R., & Earle, R. W. (2008). *Essentials of strength training and conditioning* (3rd ed.). Champaign, IL: Human Kinetics.

Graham, J. E., Boatwright, J. D., Hunskor, M. J., & Howell, D. C. (2003). Effect of active vs. passive recovery on repeat suicide run time. *Journal of Strength and Conditioning Research, 17*(2), 338–341.

Hoffman, J. R., Epstein, S., Einbinder, M., & Weinstein, Y. (2000). A comparison between the Wingate anaerobic power test to both vertical jump and line drill tests in basketball players. *Journal of Strength and Conditioning Research, 14*(3), 261–264.

Montgomery, P. G., Pyne, D. B., Hopkins, W. F., & Minahan, C. L. (2008). Seasonal progression and variability of repeated-effort line-drill performance elite junior basketball players. *Journal of Sports Sciences, 26*(5), 543–550.

Semenick, D. (1984). Anaerobic testing: Practical applications. *National Strength and Conditioning Association Journal, 6*(5), 45, 70–73.

Semenick, D. (1990). Tests and measurements: The line drill test. *National Strength and Conditioning Association Journal, 12*(2), 47–49.

■ TRIPLE 120-METER (131-YARD) SHUTTLE TEST

Objective: Measure anaerobic capacity and recovery

Age Range: High school to college age; this test is designed for rugby players, but can be utilized for other similar athletes

Equipment Needed:

1. Open grass field
2. Four cones
3. Two stopwatches

Additional Personnel Needed: Two test assistants

Setup:

1. A 3-meter (3.2-yard)-wide test corridor that is 10 meters (10.9 yards) long is created (**Figure 9-4**).
2. A test assistant is placed at line B. The test administrator and remaining test assistant remain at line A.
3. The test performer lines up behind line A.
4. The test performer may practice the protocol (described below) at partial

speed. The test performer may need to practice the ground sequence.

Administration and Directions:

1. On the test administrator's "go" command, the test performer *sprints* from line A to line B (refer to Figure 9-4).
2. When the test performer arrives at line B, he or she drops to the ground, touching the ground with the chest, and performs the following ground sequence.
   a. The test performer rolls onto the back so that both shoulders touch the ground. The test performer rolls to either the right or the left.
   b. The test performer then rolls back in the opposite direction so that the chest touches the ground. For example, if the test performer initially rolled to the right, he or she rolls back to the left.
   c. The test performer then rolls in the opposite direction he or she initially

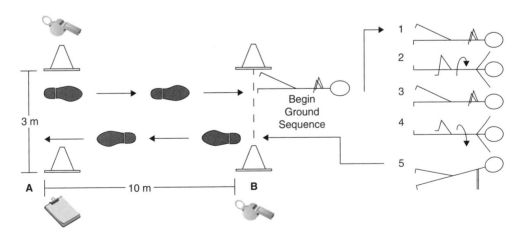

Figure 9-4   Triple 120-Meter Shuttle Test Setup and Administration

did while touching the ground with both shoulders. For example, if the test performer initially rolled to the right, now he or she rolls to the left.

   d. The test performer then rolls back in the opposite direction so that the chest touches the ground.

   e. The test performer's final position after the ground sequence should be the same approximate position as when he or she first touched the ground with the chest.

3. The test performer then *sprints* back to line A and places *both feet beyond* line A.

4. The test performer then turns and *sprints* back to line B, but needs to place only *one foot behind* line B.

5. The test performer then *sprints* back to line A and places *both feet beyond* line A.

6. This 40-meter (43.7-yard) sequence is repeated two additional times. A distance of 120 meters (131 yards) is traversed during each shuttle.

7. At the conclusion of the first shuttle, the time is recorded, and the test performer is given 1 minute to recover.

8. The test performer may walk, stretch, and consume fluids between shuttles, but should remain alert for the start of the next shuttle.

9. After the recovery period, the test performer begins the second shuttle in the same manner as the first.

10. Three shuttles are performed.

11. One complete trial is performed.

Scoring:

1. If the test performer completes any part of the test protocol incorrectly, then the trial is stopped, considered invalid, and restarted.

2. The test performer should understand how to complete the ground sequence properly *before* this test is performed. A test performer who restarts this test several times may have a relatively poor score. The test assistant who is standing at line B may give some verbal reminders and cues to the test performer during the ground sequence.

3. Each shuttle time is recorded.

4. The final score can be recorded as the best overall time or the average of the three times.

Checklist: The test performer must

1. Understand how (and practice) performing the ground sequence before the test is begun

2. Place both feet beyond line A upon each return

3. Sprint between the lines during each shuttle

4. Actively recover between shuttles

Reference

Holloway, K. M., Meir, R. A., Brooks, L. O., & Phillips, C. J. (2008). The triple-120 meter shuttle test: A sport-specific test for assessing anaerobic endurance fitness in rugby league players. *Journal of Strength and Conditioning Research, 22*(2), 633–639.

■ 40-METER MAXIMAL SHUTTLE RUN (40-M MST) TEST

Objective: Measure anaerobic capacity and recovery

Age Range: High school to college age

Equipment Needed:

1. Stopwatch
2. Open gym floor, field, or similar surface
3. Six cones or a roll of tape
4. Tape measure

Additional Personnel Needed: Two test assistants

Setup:

1. Three parallel lines are created with cones or tape 10 meters (10.9 yards) apart (**Figure 9-5**).
2. The test administrator stands perpendicular to line A, with one test assistant standing perpendicular to line B and the other perpendicular to line C.
3. The test performer lines up behind line A facing line B.

Administration and Directions:

1. On the test administrator's "go" command, the test performer *sprints* from line A toward line B until one foot is *beyond* line B (refer to Figure 9-5).
2. The test performer then turns around and *sprints* past line A to line C until one foot is *beyond* line C.
3. The test performer then turns around and *sprints* past line A.
4. A distance of 40 meters (43.7 yards) is traversed during each shuttle.
5. At the conclusion of the first shuttle, the test performer is given 20 seconds to recover.
6. The test performer may walk, stretch, and consume fluids between shuttles, but should remain alert for the start of the next shuttle.

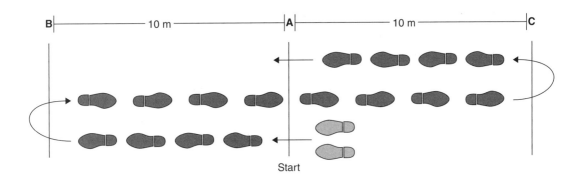

Figure 9-5 40-Meter Maximal Shuttle Run Test Setup and Administration

7. After the 20-second recovery period, the test performer begins the next shuttle in the same manner as the first.
8. The test performer performs the same protocol seven more times. A total of eight 40-meter (43.7-yard) shuttles are performed.
9. One complete trial is performed.

Scoring:

1. Each shuttle is timed and recorded.
2. The closer the times of the last two trials are to the times of the first two trials, the better the test performer's anaerobic capacity.
3. The average of the eight times is recorded as the final score.
4. The percentage decrement can be calculated and recorded. (Total sprint time = sum of sprint times from all sprints. Ideal sprint time = number of sprints × fastest sprint time.)

$$\text{fatigue \%} = 100 \times (\text{total sprint time} \div \text{ideal sprint time}) - 100$$

Checklist: The test performer must

1. Understand how to run the course
2. Touch each line with the foot before changing direction
3. Sprint straight during each trial
4. Actively recover between shuttles

References

Baker, J., Ramsbottom, R., & Hazeldine, R. (1993). Maximal shuttle running over 40m as a measure of anaerobic performance. *British Journal of Sports Medicine, 27*(4), 228–232.

Glaister, M., Hauck, H., Abraham, C. S., Merry, K. L., Beaver, D., Woods, B., & McInnes, G. (2009). Familiarization, reliability, and comparability of a 40-m maximal shuttle run test. *Journal of Sports Sciences and Medicine, 8,* 77–82.

■ REPEATED SHUTTLE SPRINT ABILITY (RSSA) TEST

Also Known as: Running Repeated Sprint Ability (rRSA) Test and Repeated Sprint Ability (RSA) Test

Objective: Measure anaerobic capacity and recovery

Age Range: High school to college age

Equipment Needed:

1. Three stopwatches
2. Open gym floor, field, or similar surface
3. Four cones or lines
4. Tape measure

Additional Personnel Needed: Two test assistants

Setup:

1. Two cones are placed 40 meters (43.7 yards) apart, with one cone placed 10 meters (10.9 yards) behind each cone (**Figure 9-6**).
2. A test assistant stands perpendicular to line A, and the other test assistant stands perpendicular to line B.
3. The test administrator stands by line A but may move between line A and line B.
4. The test performer lines up behind line A facing line B.

Administration and Directions:

1. On the test administrator's "go" command, the test performer *sprints* from line A past line B (refer to Figure 9-6).

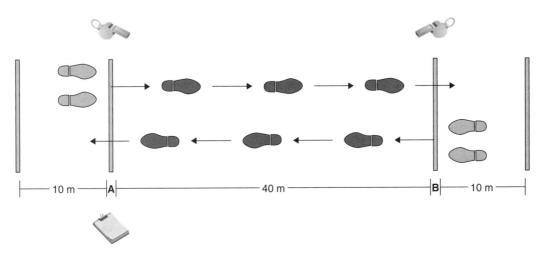

Figure 9-6   Repeated Shuttle Sprint Ability Test Setup and Administration

2. The test performer then waits at line B to *sprint* back past line A on the next "go" command.
3. The test performer has a total of 30 seconds to *sprint* to the opposite line, recover, and begin *sprinting* back to the previous line. For example, if it takes the test performer 6 seconds to *sprint* from line A to line B, he or she has 24 seconds to recover before beginning to *sprint* from line B to line A.
4. This process continues until the test performer completes six 40-meter (43.7-yard) shuttles.
5. The test performer should be encouraged to lightly walk and stretch between shuttles. The test performer should be able to jog to the cone placed 10 meters (10.9 yards) behind the line and return to the starting line during the recovery period.
6. The test administrator is responsible for keeping track of the 30-second rest time and starting each shuttle trial. Each test

assistant is responsible for timing and recording each shuttle.
7. One complete trial is performed.

Scoring:

1. Each shuttle is timed and recorded.
2. The closer the last two trials are to the first two trials, the better the test performer's anaerobic capacity.
3. The six times are averaged and recorded as the final score.
4. The percentage decrement can be calculated and recorded as well. (Total sprint time = sum of sprint times from all sprints. Ideal sprint time = number of sprints × fastest sprint time.)

fatigue % = 100 × (total sprint time ÷ ideal sprint time) – 100

Checklist: The test performer must

1. Sprint during each trial
2. Sprint through each line

3. Begin the next sprint trial 30 seconds after he or she began the previous sprint trial
4. Actively recover between shuttles

References

Aziz, A. R., & Chuan, T. E. H. (2004). Correlation between tests of running repeated sprint ability and aerobic capacity by Wingate cycling in multi-sprint sports athletes. *International Journal of Applied Sports Sciences, 16*(1), 14–22.

Aziz, A. R., Mukherjee, S., Chia, M. Y. H., & Teh, K. C. (2008). Validity of the running repeated sprint ability test among playing positions and level of competitiveness in trained soccer players. *International Journal of Sports Medicine, 29,* 833–838.

Bangsbo, J., Mohr, M., Poulsen, A., Perez-Gomez, J., & Krustrup, P. (2006). Training and testing the elite athlete. *Journal of Exercise Science and Fitness, 4*(1), 1–14.

Dawson, B., Fitzsimons, M., & Ward, D. (1993). The relationship of repeated sprint ability to aerobic power and performance measures of anaerobic work capacity and power. *Australian Journal of Science and Medicine in Sport, 25*(4), 88–93.

Ferrari Bravo, D., Impellizzeri, F. M., Rampinini, E., Castagna, C., Bishop, D., & Wisloff, U. (2008). Sprint vs. interval training in football. *International Journal of Sports Medicine, 29,* 668–671.

Fitzsimons, M., Dawson, B., Ward, D., & Wilkinson, A. (1993). Cycling and running tests of repeated sprint ability. *Australian Journal of Science and Medicine in Sport, 25*(4), 82–87.

Impellizzeri, F. M., Rampinini, E., Castagna, C., Bishop, D., Bravo, D. F., Tibaudi, A., & Wisloff, U. (2008). Validity of a repeated-sprint test for football. *International Journal of Sports Medicine, 29,* 899–905.

Keough, J. W. L., Weber, C. L., & Dalton, C. T. (2003). Evaluation of anthropometric, physiological, and skill-related tests for talent identification in female field hockey. *Canadian Journal of Applied Physiology, 28*(3), 397–409.

Spencer, M., Bishop, D., Dawson, B., & Goodman, C. (2005). Physiological and metabolic responses of repeated-sprint activities: Specific to field-based team sports. *Sports Medicine, 35*(12), 1025–1044.

Wadley, G., & Le Rossignol, P. (1998). The relationship between repeated sprint ability and the aerobic and anaerobic energy systems. *Journal of Science and Medicine in Sport, 1*(2), 100–110.

■ REPEATED 220-YARD (201-METER) SPRINT TEST

Objective: Measure anaerobic capacity and recovery

Age Range: High school to college age

Equipment Needed:

1. Two stopwatches
2. Standard outdoor track

Additional Personnel Needed: Test assistant

Setup:

1. Two start/finish lines are created on the track at the middle of each straightaway (**Figure 9-7**).
2. The test administrator is placed at one start/finish line, and the test assistant is placed at the opposite start finish line.

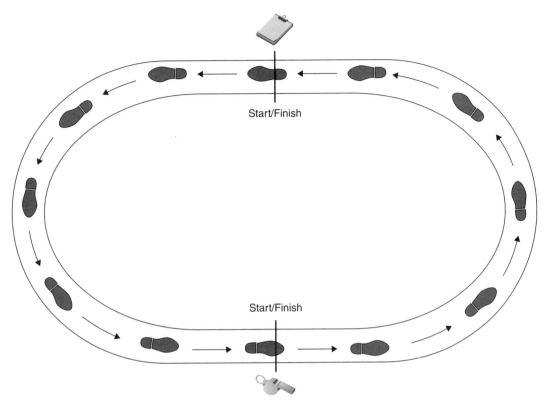

Start/Finish

Start/Finish

Figure 9-7   Repeated 200-Yard Sprint Test Setup and Administration

3. The test performer starts behind one of the start/finish lines.

Administration and Directions:

1. On the test administrator's (or test assistant's) "go" command, the test performer *sprints* around the track and past the opposite start/finish line (refer to Figure 9-7).
2. Once the test performer completes the trial, he or she is given rest at a ratio of 1:3 (i.e., 30-second sprint = 90 seconds of rest) before another *sprint* trial is performed.
3. The test performer may walk, stretch, and consume fluids between sprint trials, but should remain alert for the start of the next sprint.

4. After the rest period, the test performer begins the second sprint in the same manner as the first.
5. A total of 12 sprints are completed.
6. The test administrator or test assistant on the opposite side from where the test performer starts the sprint is the timer for that particular sprint, and the test administrator/assistant at the line where the test performer begins the sprint drops his or her arm when the test performer is given the "go" command.
7. One complete trial is performed.

Scoring:

1. Each sprint is timed and recorded.
2. The average time of the 12 sprints is recorded as the final score.

Checklist: The test performer must

1. Maximally sprint through the finish line during each trial
2. Actively recover between shuttles

Reference

Semenick, D. (1984). Anaerobic testing: Practical applications. *National Strength and Conditioning Association Journal, 6*(5), 45, 70–73.

■ 5-METER (5.5-YARD) MULTIPLE SHUTTLE TEST

Objective: Measure anaerobic endurance

Age Range: High school to college age

Equipment Needed:

1. Two stopwatches
2. Six cones
3. Tape measure
4. Open, flat running surface

Additional Personnel Needed: Two test assistants

Setup:

1. The six cones are placed in a straight line 5 meters (5.5 yards) apart (**Figure 9-8**).
2. One test assistant is positioned on the course to document how far the test performer runs and to ensure he or she performs the test sequence correctly.
3. The test administrator and the other test assistant stand perpendicular to the starting line.
4. The test performer may practice the protocol (described below) at partial speed.
5. The test performer begins behind the starting line (cone A).

Administration and Directions:

1. On the test administrator's "go" command, the test performer *sprints* from cone A to cone B and touches the ground adjacent to the cone (refer to Figure 9-8).
2. The test performer then *sprints* back to cone A and touches the ground adjacent to the cone.
3. The test performer then *sprints* to cone C and touches the ground adjacent to the cone before returning to cone A.
4. The test performer continues to run the course continuously for 30 seconds.
5. At the conclusion of the first shuttle, the time is recorded, and the test performer is given 35 seconds to recover.
6. The test performer may walk, stretch, and consume fluids between shuttles, but should remain alert for the start of the next shuttle. The test performer should use this time to get ready behind line A before the next shuttle.
7. After the rest period, the test performer begins the second shuttle in the same manner as the first.
8. Six shuttles are performed.
9. One complete trial is performed.

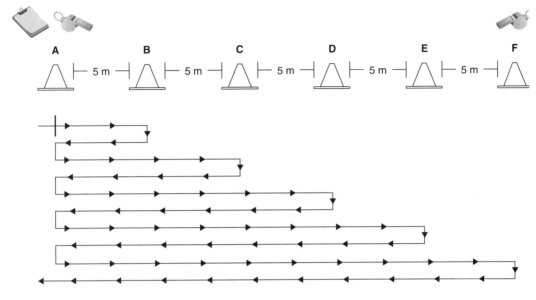

Figure 9-8   5-Meter Multiple Shuttle Test Setup and Administration

Scoring:

1. If a test performer completes any portion of the test incorrectly, the trial is stopped, considered invalid, and restarted.
2. When the test administrator gives the "stop" command, the test assistant who is placed on the course marks where the test performer's *body* is.
3. The test administrator adds the total distance the test performer traverses during each 30-second sprint trial to the nearest 2.5 meters (2.7 yards).
4. The final score is recorded as one of the following. (Shuttles 1 and 2 distances are the farthest distances traversed. Shuttles 5 and 6 distances are the shortest distances traversed.)

peak distance = greatest distance traversed during a 30-second shuttle

total distance = total distance traversed during one complete trial

delta distance = difference between the longest and shortest shuttle distances

fatigue index = [(shuttle 1 distance + shuttle 2 distance) − (shuttle 5 distance + shuttle 6 distance)] ÷ [(shuttle 1 distance + shuttle 2 distance) ÷ 2] × 100

Checklist: The test performer must

1. Understand how to run the course
2. Maximally sprint during the test
3. Begin the subsequent sprint trial 35 seconds after completing the previous sprint trial
4. Actively recover between shuttles

Reference

Boddington, M. K., Lambert, M. I., St. Clair Gibson, A., & Noakes, T. D. Reliability of a 5-m multiple shuttle test. *Journal of Sports Sciences, 19*, 223–228.

Agility Testing

Agility is the ability to stop, start, and change the direction of the body (or body parts) rapidly and in a controlled manner. Agility typically signifies a change in movement velocity or performing locomotion movements other than linear sprinting. Components of agility include strength, speed, coordination, and dynamic balance. For many athletic endeavors, agility is the single most important parameter of how well an individual will perform in a given sport or activity.

The test administrator must instruct and ensure that all test performers properly warm up and stretch before any agility test is conducted. If the agility test has multiple trials, the test performer should be instructed and encouraged to properly rest and recover between trials by walking, stretching, and consuming fluids. Agility tests should be conducted when the test performer is well rested. All agility test performers should wear proper footwear that will provide good traction for the surface the test is administered on. The test administrator should choose a non-slip surface for any agility test. The test surface should be similar to the surface on which the test performer will conduct the planned physical activity. Agility tests should not be conducted in order to elicit fatigue or be conducted when a test performer is fatigued.

■ RIGHT BOOMERANG RUN TEST

Objective: Measure running agility

Age Range: 10 to college age

Equipment Needed:

1. Stopwatch
2. Tape measure
3. Chair (or a similar obstacle)
4. Four cones
5. Large floor area

Additional Personnel Needed: None

Setup:

1. A start/finish line is created and marked with a cone.
2. A chair (or similar obstacle) is placed 17 feet (5.2 meters) from the starting line.
3. Three additional cones are placed 15 feet (4.5 meters) from the chair on the remaining three sides (**Figure 10-1**).
4. The test performer may practice running the course (described below) at partial speed.
5. The test performer lines up on the *left* of the start/finish line facing the chair.

Administration and Directions:

1. On the test administrator's "go" command, the test performer *sprints* to the chair, makes a quarter turn *right*, and runs around the cone back to the chair, where another quarter *right* turn is made (refer to Figure 10-1).
2. The test performer continues this process of making quarter *right* turns around the chair until *sprinting* through the start/finish line.
3. The test performer should walk and stretch between trials.
4. Three trials are performed.

Scoring:

1. If a test performer executes any portion of the test incorrectly, the trial is stopped, considered invalid, and restarted.
2. A penalty of 0.1 seconds is added to the test performer's score each time he or she touches an obstacle.
3. The best time is recorded as the final score.

Checklist: The test performer must

1. Understand how to run the course (test performer may need to jog or walk the course to become accustomed to the pattern)
2. Sprint around the chair and cones without touching any
3. Actively recover between trials

Note: This test may be performed as a left boomerang run. The protocol is identical, except the test performer will start on the right of the start/finish line and make quarter turns to the left instead of the right.

References

Gates, D. P., & Sheffield, R. P. (1940). Test of change of direction as measurement of different kinds of motor ability in boys of 7th, 8th, and 9th Grades. *Research Quarterly, 11,* 136–147.

Johnson, B. L., & Nelson, J. K. (1986). *Practical measurements for evaluation in physical education* (4th ed.). New York: MacMillan.

Miller, D. K. (2006). *Measurement by the physical educator: Why and how* (5th ed.). New York: McGraw-Hill.

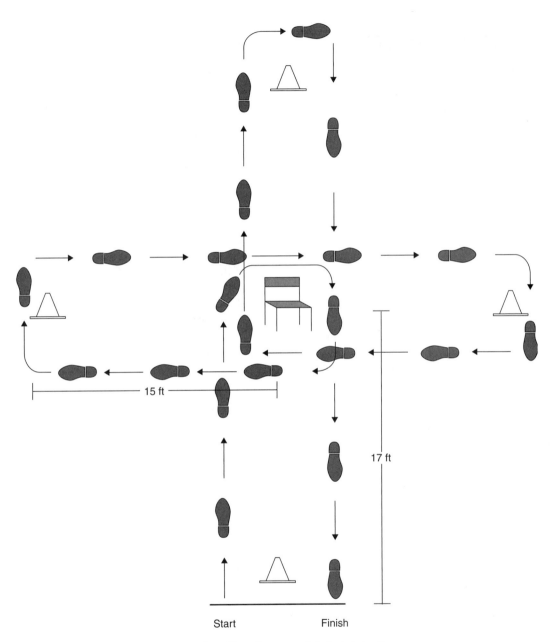

Figure 10-1   Right Boomerang Run Test Setup and Administration

■ SIDESTEPPING TEST

Objective: Measure lateral movement agility, endurance, and speed

Age Range: 9 to adult

Equipment Needed:

1. Stopwatch
2. Tape measure
3. Floor tape
4. Large floor area

Additional Personnel Needed: Test assistant

Setup:

1. The floor tape is used to create two parallel lines on the floor 12 feet (3.6 meters) apart, as measured from the *inside* of the lines (**Figure 10-2**).
2. The test performer may practice running the course (described below) at partial speed.
3. The test performer starts with the body inside the lines, with one foot placed on a line.

Administration and Directions:

1. On the test administrator's "go" command, the test performer steps laterally toward the opposite line, *leading with the foot nearest to the line being approached* (refer to Figure 10-2).
2. The test performer continues until the lead foot *touches or crosses* the line.

3. Once the opposite line is touched or crossed, the test performer changes directions and returns to the opposite line in the same manner, *while facing the same direction.*
4. This protocol is repeated continuously for 30 seconds.
5. One trial is performed.

Scoring:

1. Each time the test performer's foot touches or crosses a line is counted as 1 point.
2. If the test performer's foot does not touch or cross a line, no point is given.
3. The total points earned are recorded as the final score.

Checklist: The test performer must

1. Face the same direction during the test at all times
2. Not cross the feet or legs during the test
3. Step with the foot closest to the line being approached before moving the other foot

Reference

Miller, D. K. (2006). *Measurement by the physical educator: Why and how* (5th ed.). New York: McGraw-Hill.

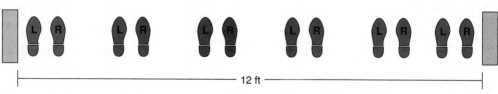

|———————————— 12 ft ————————————|

Figure 10-2   Sidestepping Test Setup and Administration

■ EDGREN SIDE STEP TEST

Objective: Measure lateral agility

Age Range: Middle school to college age

Equipment Needed:

1. Stopwatch
2. Tape measure
3. Floor tape
4. Flat floor at least 15 feet long and 10 feet wide (4.5 meters long and 3 meters wide)

Additional Personnel Needed: Test assistant

Setup:

1. Five strips of tape are placed parallel on the floor 3 feet (0.9 meters) apart (**Figure 10-3**).
2. The test performer straddles the center line.
3. The test performer may practice performing this test (described below) at partial speed.
4. The test administrator and test assistant stand on opposite sides of the test performer, front and back.

Administration and Directions:

1. On the test administrator's "go" command, the test performer shuffles to the *right* (leading with the foot closest to the line being approached) until the right foot either *touches or crosses* the farthest line (refer to Figure 10-3).

2. The test performer then shuffles to the *left* until the left foot either *touches or crosses* the farthest line.
3. The test performer continues this protocol continuously for 10 seconds.
4. The test performer should walk and stretch between trials.
5. Two trials are performed.

Scoring:

1. Each time the test performer's body crosses a line or foot contacts (or crosses) the outermost line is counted as 1 point.
2. A 1-point penalty is given each time the test performer's feet cross and each time the test performer does not successfully touch (or cross) the outermost line before changing directions.
3. It is helpful to have the test assistant count the penalties while the test administrator counts the earned points.
4. The penalty points are subtracted from the number of points earned and recorded as the final score.

final score = correct foot contacts
– penalty points

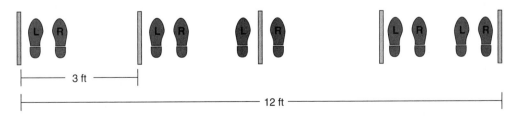

|← 3 ft →|

|← 12 ft →|

Figure 10-3   Edgren Side Step Test Setup and Administration

Checklist: The test performer must

1. Understand how to perform the test
2. Not cross the feet
3. Lead with the foot closest to the line that is being approached
4. Actively recover between shuttles

References

Baechle, T. R., & Earle, R. W. (2008). *Essentials of strength training and conditioning* (3rd ed.). Champaign, IL: Human Kinetics.

Coaches roundtable: Testing for football. (1983). *National Strength and Conditioning Association Journal, 5*(5), 12–19.

Edgren, H. (1932). An experiment in the testing ability and progress in basketball. *Research Quarterly, 3*(1), 159–171.

Farlinger, C. M., Kruisselbrink, L. D., & Fowles, J. R. (2007). Relationships to skating performance in competitive hockey players. *Journal of Strength and Conditioning Research, 21*(3), 915–922.

Semenick, D. (1981). Conditioning program: Testing and evaluation. *National Strength and Conditioning Association Journal, 3*(2), 8–9.

■ SEMO AGILITY TEST

Objective: Measure running agility while moving the body forward, backward, and sideways

Age Range: High school to college age

Equipment Needed:

1. Stopwatch
2. Lined basketball free-throw lane
3. Four cones

Additional Personnel Needed: None

Setup:

1. One cone is placed in each corner of the free-throw lane of a basketball court. If a free-throw lane is not available, a 12- by 19-foot (3.6- by 5.8-meter) rectangle is created on an acceptable surface (**Figure 10-4**).
2. The test performer may practice running the course (described below) at partial speed.

3. The test performer lines up at point A, facing the free-throw line.

Administration and Directions:

1. On the test administrator's "go" command, the test performer *sidesteps left* to the outside of point B (refer to Figure 10-4).
2. The test performer then *backpedals* from point B to point D, *passing outside* point D. The test performer should be facing point A.
3. The test performer then *sprints* forward to point A, *passing around* the cone.
4. The test performer then backpedals from point A to point C, *passing outside* point C. The test performer should be facing point B.
5. The test performer then *sprints* to point B, *passing around* the cone.
6. The test performer then *sidesteps right* to the start/finish line at point A.

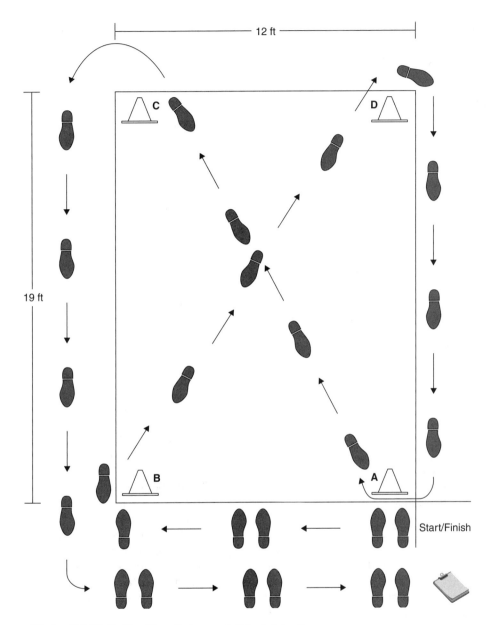

Figure 10-4 SEMO Agility Test Setup and Administration

7. The test performer should walk and stretch between trials.
8. Two trials are performed.

Scoring:

1. If a test performer executes any portion of the test incorrectly, the trial is stopped, considered invalid, and restarted.
2. The best time is recorded as the final score.

Checklist: The test performer must

1. Understand how to run the course
2. Run around each cone

3. Backpedal and sidestep in a straight line
4. Actively recover between shuttles

References

Johnson, B. L., & Nelson, J. K. (1986). *Practical measurements for evaluation in physical education* (4th ed.). New York: MacMillan.

Kirby, R. F. (1971, June). A simple test of agility. *Coach and Athlete*, 30–31.

Miller, D. K. (2006). *Measurement by the physical educator: Why and how* (5th ed.). New York: McGraw-Hill.

■ AAHPERD SHUTTLE RUN TEST

Objective: Measure running agility

Age Range: 9 to college age

Equipment Needed:

1. Stopwatch
2. Tape measure
3. Floor tape
4. Two objects that can be easily grasped and run with (i.e., board erasers or wood blocks)
5. Large, flat running surface

Additional Personnel Needed: None

Setup:

1. The floor tape is used to create two parallel lines on the floor 30 feet (9.1 meters) apart (**Figure 10-5**).
2. The two objects are placed on the floor just across the line that is opposite the start/finish line. If objects are not available, the test performer can touch the lines instead of grasping objects.

3. The test performer lines up behind the start/finish line, facing the opposite line.

Administration and Directions:

1. On the test administrator's "go" command, the test performer *sprints* from the start/finish line toward the opposite line, stops, and picks up one object (refer to Figure 10-5).
2. The test performer then *sprints* back to the start/finish line, stops, and *places* the object on the floor.
3. The test performer repeats this protocol for the second object.
4. The test performer should walk and stretch between trials.
5. Two trials are performed.

Scoring:

1. If the test performer executes any portion of this test incorrectly, the trial is stopped, considered invalid, and restarted.
2. The best time is recorded as the final score.

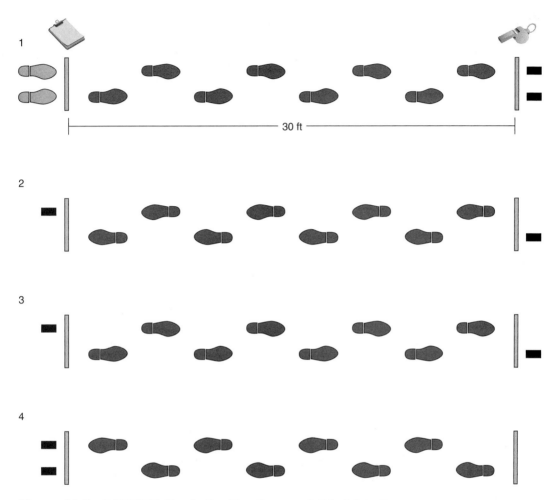

Figure 10-5 AAHPERD Shuttle Run Test Setup and Administration

Checklist: The test performer must

1. Not throw or drop the objects when returning to the start/finish line
2. Sprint during each shuttle
3. Actively recover between shuttles

References

American Association for Health, Physical Education, Recreation, and Dance (AAHPERD).

(1976). *AAHPER youth fitness test manual.* Washington, DC: AAHPERD.

Brodie, D. A. (1996). *A reference manual for human performance measurement in the field of physical education and sports sciences.* Lewiston, NY: Edwin Mellen Press.

Gates, D. P., & Sheffield, R. P. (1940. Test of change of direction as measurement of different kinds of motor ability in boys of 7th, 8th, and 9th Grades. *Research Quarterly, 11,* 136–147.

McSwegin, P., Pemberton, C., Petray, C., & Going, S. (1989). *Physical best: The AAHPERD guide to physical fitness education and assessment.* Reston, VA: AAHPERD.

Miller, D. K. (2006). *Measurement by the physical educator: Why and how* (5th ed.). New York: McGraw-Hill.

Safrit, M. J. (1995). *Complete guide to youth fitness testing.* Champaign, IL: Human Kinetics.

■ BARROW ZIGZAG RUN TEST

Objective: Measure running agility

Age Range: Middle school to college age

Equipment Needed:

1. Stopwatch
2. Tape measure
3. Five cones
4. Large, flat running surface

Additional Personnel Needed: None

Setup:

1. One cone is placed in each corner of a 10- by 16-foot (3- by 4.9-meter) rectangle (**Figure 10-6**).
2. The fifth cone is placed in the center of the rectangle.
3. The test performer may practice running the course (described below) at partial speed.
4. The test performer begins in the lower right-hand corner at point A, facing point B.

Administration and Directions:

1. On the test administrator's "go" command, the test performer *sprints* toward the center cone, makes a *half turn right*, and *sprints* to point B (refer to Figure 10-6).
2. The test performer then *turns left* around point B and *sprints* toward point C.
3. The test performer then *turns left* around point C and *sprints* toward the center

cone, makes a *half turn right*, and *sprints* to point D.

4. The test performer then *turns left* around point D and *sprints* toward point A.
5. The test performer then *turns left* around point A and completes two additional laps on the course until three laps are completed.
6. The test performer should walk and stretch between trials.
7. Two trials are performed.

Scoring:

1. If a test performer executes any portion of this test incorrectly, the trial is stopped, considered invalid, and restarted.
2. The best time is recorded as the final score.

Checklist: The test performer must
1. Understand how to run the course
2. Sprint around each cone without touching it
3. Understand that each trial consists of three laps
4. Actively recover between shuttles

References

Barrow, H. M. (1954). Tests of motor ability for college men. *Research Quarterly, 25,* 253–260.

Miller, D. K. (2006). *Measurement by the physical educator: Why and how* (5th ed.). New York: McGraw-Hill.

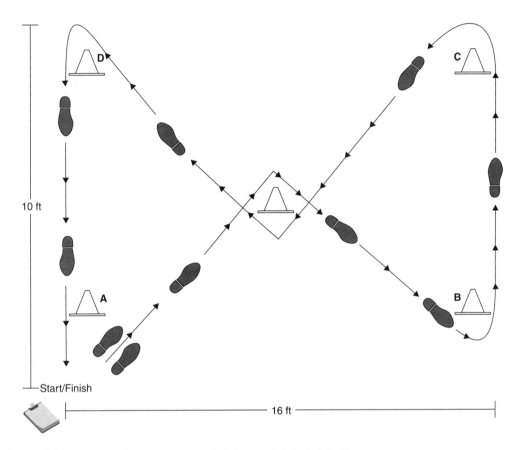

Figure 10-6   Barrow Zigzag Run Test Setup and Administration

---

■ T-TEST

Objective: Measure four-directional agility and body control

Age Range: High school to college age

Equipment Needed:

1. Stopwatch
2. Tape measure
3. Four cones
4. Large, flat running surface

Additional Personnel Needed: One test assistant

Setup:

1. Two cones are placed 10 yards (9.1 meters) apart on the floor in a straight line.
2. The third cone is placed in the center of the first two cones, with the fourth cone

placed 10 yards (9.1 meters) away from the center cone in a straight line with the third cone.

3. The course should be in the shape of a T (**Figure 10-7**).

4. The test performer may practice running the course (described below) at partial speed.

5. The test performer lines up on the *left* side of point A, facing point B.

Administration and Directions:

1. On the test administrator's "go" command, the test performer *sprints* from point A to point B and touches the *base* of the cone with the *right* hand (refer to Figure 10-7).

2. Then, facing the same direction and not crossing the feet, the test performer *shuffles* to the left to point C and touches the *base* of the cone with the *left* hand.

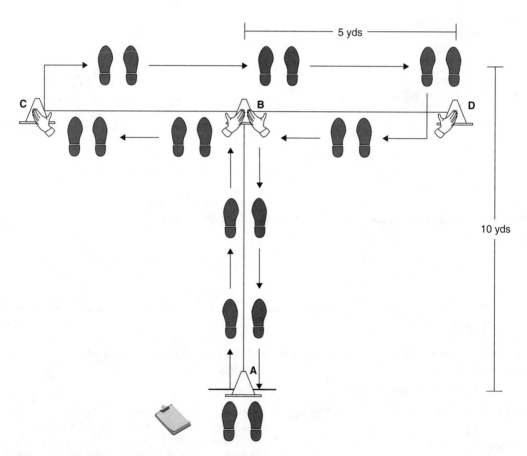

Figure 10-7 T-Test Setup and Administration

3. Then, facing the same direction and not crossing the feet, the test performer *shuffles* to the right past point B to point D and touches the *base* of the cone with the *right* hand.
4. Then, facing the same direction and not crossing the feet, the test performer *shuffles* to point B and touches the *base* of the cone with the *left* hand.
5. Then, facing the same direction, the test performer *backpedals* past point A.
6. A test assistant, another test performer, or an exercise mat should be positioned behind point A to catch a test performer who may fall while finishing the course.
7. The test performer should walk and stretch between trials.
8. Two trials are performed.

Scoring:

1. If a test performer executes any portion of the test incorrectly, the trial is stopped, considered invalid, and restarted.
2. The best time is recorded as the final score.

Checklist: The test performer must

1. Understand how to run the course
2. Not cross the feet when shuffling

3. Face the same direction during the test
4. Actively recover between shuttles

References

Baechle, T. R., & Earle, R. W. (2008). *Essentials of strength training and conditioning* (3rd ed.). Champaign, IL: Human Kinetics.

McMillian, D. J., Moore, J. H., Hatler, B. S., & Taylor, D. C. (2006). Dynamic vs. static-stretching warm *up:* The effect on power and agility performance. *Journal of Strength and Conditioning Research, 20*(3), 492–499.

Miller, M. G., Herniman, J. J., Ricard, M. D., Cheatham, C. C., & Michael, T. J. (2006). The effects of a 6-week plyometric training program on agility. *Journal of Sports Science and Medicine, 5,* 456–465.

Pauole, K., Madole, K., Garhammer, J., Lacourse, M., & Rozenek, R. (2000). Reliability and validity of the T-test as a measure of agility, leg power, and leg speed in college-aged men and women. *Journal of Strength and Conditioning Research, 14*(4), 443–450.

Semenick, D. (1990). Tests and measurements: The T-test. *NSCA Journal, 12*(1), 36–37.

■ ILLINOIS AGILITY TEST

Objective: Measure running agility while cutting and weaving

Age Range: 10 to college age

Equipment Needed:

1. Stopwatch
2. Tape measure
3. Eight cones
4. Large, flat running surface

Additional Personnel Needed: None

Setup:

1. A 5- by 10-meter (5.5- by 10.9-yard) box is created with four cones.
2. The remaining four cones are placed 1.6 meters (5.2 feet) apart in a straight line down the center of the box (**Figure 10-8**).

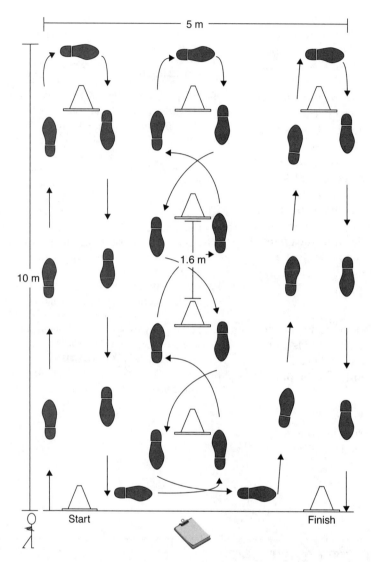

Figure 10-8   Illinois Agility Test Setup and Administration

3. The test performer may practice running the course (described below) at partial speed.
4. The test performer lies on the stomach, with the hands by the shoulders and the head at the starting line at point A, facing the opposite line.

Administration and Directions:

1. On the test administrator's "go" command, the test performer *sprints* from the starting position to the opposite line, touches the line with a foot, and then

sprints back to touch the starting line (refer to Figure 10-8).

2. The test performer then *weaves* through the center cones, by *initially going left* (then right) to the opposite line (touching the line).

3. The test performer then *weaves* back through the center cones to the opposite line (touching the line).

4. The test performer then *sprints* to the opposite line (on the other side of the center cones), touches the line, and *sprints* through the start/finish line.

5. The test performer should walk and stretch between trials.

6. Two trials are performed.

Scoring:

1. If a test performer executes any portion of the test incorrectly, or knocks over a cone, the trial is stopped, considered invalid, and restarted.

2. The best time is recorded as the final score.

Checklist: The test performer must

1. Understand how to run the course

2. Touch each end line and weave between the center cones

3. Start the test lying on the stomach

4. Actively recover between shuttles

References

Draper, J. A., & Lancaster, M. G. (1985). The 505 test: A test for agility in the horizontal plane. *Australian Journal of Science and Medicine in Sport, 17*(1), 15–18.

Getchell, B., Mikesky, A. E., & Mikesky, K. N. (1998). *Physical fitness: A way of life* (5th ed.). Boston: Allyn and Bacon.

Keough, J. W. L., Weber, C. L., & Dalton, C. T. (2003). Evaluation of anthropometric, physiological, and skill-related tests for talent identification in female field hockey. *Canadian Journal of Applied Physiology, 28*(3), 397–409.

Miller, M. G., Herniman, J. J., Ricard, M. D., Cheatham, C. C., & Michael, T. J. (2006). The effects of a 6-week plyometric training program on agility. *Journal of Sports Science and Medicine, 5*, 456–465.

Roozen, M. (2004). Illinois agility test. *NSCA's Performance Training Journal, 3*(5), 5–6.

Sheppard, J. M., & Young, W. B. (2006). Agility literature review: Classifications, training and testing. *Journal of Sports Sciences, 24*(9), 919–932.

Svensson, M., & Drust, B. (2005). Testing soccer players. *Journal of Sports Sciences, 23*(6), 601–618.

■ UP AND BACK (UAB) AGILITY TEST

Also Known as: 15-Meter Shuttle Test

Objective: Measure running agility

Age Range: Child to adult

Equipment Needed:

1. Stopwatch
2. Tape measure
3. Two cones
4. Large, flat running surface

Additional Personnel Needed: Test assistant

Setup:

1. A course is created where the two cones are spaced 15 meters (16.4 yards) apart (**Figure 10-9**).

2. The test assistant stands perpendicular to the non-starting cone.

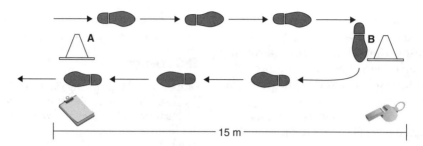

Figure 10-9 Up and Back Agility Test Setup and Administration

3. The test administrator stands perpendicular to the starting cone.
4. The test performer lines up behind cone A.

Administration and Directions:

1. On the test administrator's "go" command, the test performer *sprints* from cone A and places one foot behind cone B (refer to Figure 10-9).
2. The test performer then immediately pivots at cone B and *sprints* back past cone A.
3. The test performer should walk and stretch between trials.
4. Three trials are performed.

Scoring:

1. If the test performer does not place one foot behind cone B, the trial is stopped, considered invalid, and restarted.
2. The test administrator starts timing on the "go" command and stops timing when the test performer sprints through cone A.

3. The best time is recorded as the final score.

Checklist: The test performer must

1. Understand how to run the course
2. Place one foot beyond cone B
3. Sprint the entire course
4. Actively recover between shuttles

References

Castagna, C., Impellizzeri, F. M., Rampinini, E., D'Ottavio, S. D., & Manzi, V. (2008). The yo-yo intermittent recovery test in basketball players. *Journal of Science and Medicine in Sport, 11,* 202–208.

Draper, J. A., & Lancaster, M. G. (1985). The 505 test: A test for agility in the horizontal plane. *Australian Journal of Science and Medicine in Sport, 17*(1), 15–18.

■ 505 AGILITY TEST

Objective: Measure agility of an athlete while already at running speed and while making a 180° turn; additionally, linear acceleration is partially tested

Age Range: High school to college age

Equipment Needed:

1. Stopwatch (or an electronic timing system)
2. Tape measure
3. Large, flat running surface

Additional Personnel Needed: None

Setup:

1. A course is created that is 15 meters (16.4 yards) long, with one section being 10 meters (10.9 yards) long and the other section 5 meters (5.5 meters) long (**Figure 10-10**).
2. The test administrator stands at line B.
3. The test performer may practice running the course (described below) at partial speed.
4. The test performer lines up behind line A, facing line B.

Administration and Directions:

1. On the test administrator's "go" command, the test performer *sprints*

from line A through line B to line C (refer to Figure 10-10).

2. The test performer then touches line C, pivots 180° (on their preferred foot), and then *sprints* back through line B on the return to line A.
3. The test performer should walk and stretch between trials.
4. Three trials are performed.
5. The test administrator may have the test performer complete another three trials on the non-preferred foot in the same manner for a total of six trials.

Scoring:

1. If a test performer executes any portion of the test incorrectly, the trial is stopped, considered invalid, and restarted.
2. The test administrator starts timing when the test performer initially passes through line B (on the way to line C) and stops timing when the test performer returns past line B (on the way to line A). This test was originally designed to be measured by an electronic timing system, but it can be measured using a stopwatch.

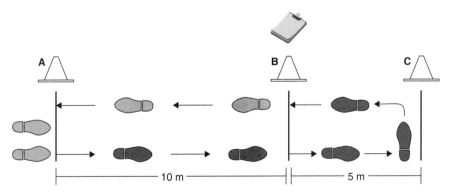

Figure 10-10   505 Agility Test Setup and Administration

3. The best time is recorded as the final score.
4. The test administrator may choose to record the test performer's best time for each foot (i.e., pivoting on the preferred and then the non-preferred foot).

Checklist: The test performer must

1. Understand how to run the course
2. Be at full speed when passing line B
3. Touch line C without significantly overstepping it
4. Sprint through line B on the way back to line A
5. Actively recover between shuttles

References

Draper, J. A., & Lancaster, M. G. (1985). The 505 test: A test for agility in the horizontal plane. *Australian Journal of Science and Medicine in Sport, 17*(1), 15–18.

Gabbett, T. J., Kelly, J. N., & Sheppard, J. M. (2008). Speed, change of direction speed, and reactive agility of rugby league players. *Journal of Strength and Conditioning Research, 22*(1), 174–181.

Gore, C. J. (2000). *Physiological tests for elite athletes.* Australian Sports Commission. Champaign, IL: Human Kinetics.

Sheppard, J. M., & Young, W. B. (2006). Agility literature review: Classifications, training and testing. *Journal of Sports Sciences, 24*(9), 919–932.

Svensson, M., & Drust, B. (2005). Testing soccer players. *Journal of Sports Sciences, 23*(6), 601–618.

■ PRO-AGILITY TEST

Also Known as: 20-Yard (22.8-Meter) Shuttle Test and 5–10–5 Test

Objective: Measure running agility, lateral speed, and coordination

Age Range: Junior high to college age

Equipment Needed:

1. Stopwatch
2. Three cones
3. Tape measure
4. Open gym floor or a lined American football field

Additional Personnel Needed: Test assistant

Setup:

1. Three parallel lines are created 5 yards (4.5 meters) apart on the floor and marked by cones. A lined American football field can be utilized as the course (**Figure 10-11**).
2. The test performer may practice performing this test (described below) at partial speed.
3. The test performer straddles the center line (line A) and assumes a 3-point stance.

Administration and Directions:

1. On the test administrator's "go" command, the test performer *sprints* from line A to the *left* and touches the line B with the foot (refer to Figure 10-11).
2. The performer then stops and *sprints* past line A to line C, touching line C with the foot.
3. The test performer then *sprints* back through line A.

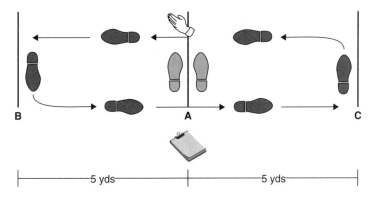

Figure 10-11 Pro-Agility Test Setup and Administration

4. The test performer should walk and stretch between trials.
5. Two trials are performed.

Scoring:

1. If the test performer executes any portion of the test incorrectly, the trial is stopped, considered invalid, and restarted.
2. The test administrator begins timing on the "go" command and stops timing when the test performer sprints through line A.
3. The best time is recorded as the final score.

Checklist: The test performer must

1. Understand how to run the course
2. Start with the body straddling the center line and in a 3-point stance
3. Touch both of the outer lines with the foot
4. Finish the test by running through line A
5. Actively recover between shuttles

References

Baechle, T. R., & Earle, R. W. (2008). *Essentials of strength training and conditioning* (3rd ed.). Champaign, IL: Human Kinetics.

Coaches roundtable: Testing for football. (1983). *National Strength and Conditioning Association Journal, 5*(5), 12–19.

Davis, D. S., Barnette, B. J., Kiger, J. T., Mirasola, J. J., & Young, S. M. (2004). Physical characteristics that predict functional performance in Division I college football players. *Journal of Strength and Conditioning Research, 18*(1), 115–120.

Greene, J. J., McGuine, T. A., Leverson, G., & Best, T. M. (1998). Anthropometric and performance measures for high school basketball players. *Journal of Athletic Training, 33*(3), 229–232.

Inside the Combine. (2008, February 20). *Chicago Tribune,* 5–7.

Kuzmits, F. E., & Adams, A. J. The NFL Combine: Does it predict performance in the National Football League? *Journal of Strength and Conditioning Research, 22*(6), 1721–1727.

McGee, K. J., & Burkett, L. N. (2003). The National Football League Combine: A reliable predictor of draft status. *Journal of Strength and Conditioning Research, 17*(1), 6–11.

Nesser, T. W., Huxel, K. C., Tincher, J. L., & Okada, T. (2008). The relationship between core stability and performance in division I football players. *Journal of Strength and Conditioning Research, 22*(6), 1750–1754.

Sierer, S. P., Battaglini, C. L., Mihalik, J. P., Shields, E. W., & Tomasini, N. T. (2008). The National Football League Combine: Performance differences between drafted and nondrafted players entering the 2004 and 2005 drafts. *Journal of Strength and Conditioning Research, 22*(1), 6–12.

■ 3-CONE DRILL

Also Known as: L-Drill/L-Run and 3-Corner Shuttle Run Test

Objective: Measure running agility

Age Range: Junior high to college age

Equipment Needed:

1. Stopwatch
2. Tape measure
3. Three cones
4. Flat running surface

Additional Personnel Needed: None

Setup:

1. Two cones are placed parallel 5 yards (4.5 meters) apart.
2. The remaining cone is placed 5 yards (4.5 meters) from one of the first two cones at a 90° angle (**Figure 10-12**).
3. The course should look like an L.
4. The test performer may practice running the course (described below) at partial speed.
5. The test performer lines up at point A, facing point B.

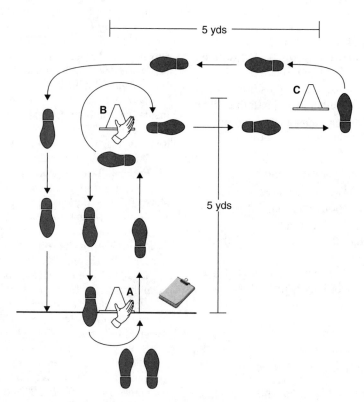

Figure 10-12   3-Cone Drill Setup and Administration

Administration and Directions:

1. On the test administrator's "go" command, the test performer *sprints* from point A to point B, touching the base of the cone with the *right* hand (refer to Figure 10-12).
2. The test performer then *sprints* back to point A, touching the base of the cone with the *right* hand.
3. The test performer then *sprints* from point A to point C, making a *clockwise* turn around point B (point B is on the right side).
4. The test performer *circles around* point C in a *counterclockwise* direction and immediately *sprints* to point A by making a *left* turn around point B.
5. The test performer should walk and stretch between trials.
6. Two trials are performed.

Scoring:

1. If the test performer knocks over any cone or executes any portion of the test incorrectly, the trial is stopped, considered invalid, and restarted.
2. The test administrator begins timing on the "go" command and stops timing when the test performer sprints through point A.
3. The best time is recorded as the final score.

Checklist: The test performer must

1. Understand how to run the course
2. Start with the body facing toward point B
3. Turn *counterclockwise* around point C
4. Finish the test by running through the finish line
5. Actively recover between shuttles

References

Coaches roundtable: Testing for football. (1983). *National Strength and Conditioning Association Journal, 5*(5), 12–19.

Gabbett, T. J., Kelly, J. N., & Sheppard, J. M. (2008). Speed, change of direction speed, and reactive agility of rugby league players. *Journal of Strength and Conditioning Research, 22*(1), 174–181.

Inside the Combine. (2008, February 20). *Chicago Tribune,* 5–7.

Kuzmits, F. E., & Adams, A. J. The NFL Combine: Does it predict performance in the National Football League? *Journal of Strength and Conditioning Research, 22*(6), 1721–1727.

McGee, K. J., & Burkett, L. N. (2003). The National Football League Combine: A reliable predictor of draft status. *Journal of Strength and Conditioning Research, 17*(1), 6–11.

Meir, R., Newton, R., Curtis, E., Fardell, M., & Butler, B. (2001). Physical fitness qualities of professional rugby league football players: Determination of positional differences. *Journal of Strength and Conditioning Research, 15*(4), 450–458.

Nesser, T. W., Huxel, K. C., Tincher, J. L., & Okada, T. (2008). The relationship between core stability and performance in division I football players. *Journal of Strength and Conditioning Research, 22*(6), 1750–1754.

Sierer, S. P., Battaglini, C. L., Mihalik, J. P., Shields, E. W., & Tomasini, N. T. (2008). The National Football League Combine: Performance differences between drafted and nondrafted players entering the 2004 and 2005 drafts. *Journal of Strength and Conditioning Research, 22*(1), 6–12.

■ NEBRASKA AGILITY RUN TEST

Objective: Measure running agility

Age Range: High school to college age

Equipment Needed:

1. Stopwatch
2. Tape measure
3. Three cones
4. Flat, open surface

Additional Personnel Needed: None

Setup:

1. Two cones are placed parallel 5 yards (4.5 meters) apart, with the third cone 5 yards (4.5 meters) away between the two cones that are parallel (**Figure 10-13**).
2. The test performer may practice performing this test (described below) at partial speed.

3. The test performer stands behind cone A, facing cone B.

Administration and Directions:

1. On the test administrator's "go" command, the test performer *sprints* from cone A *around* cone B. The test performer should round cone B by turning *right* (refer to Figure 10-13).
2. The test performer then continues *sprinting* to cone C and makes a *left* turn around cone C.
3. The test performer then *sprints* to the line where cone B is placed and touches the line with the hand.
4. The test performer then *backpedals* through the line where cones A and C are placed.

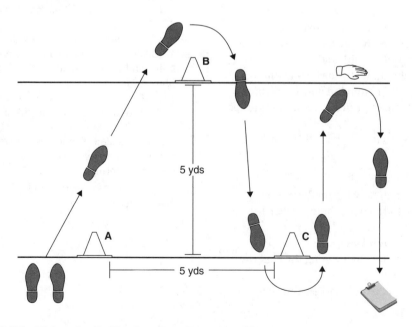

Figure 10-13 Nebraska Agility Run Test Setup and Administration

5. The test performer should walk and stretch between trials.
6. Two trials are performed.

Scoring:

1. If the test performer knocks over any cone or executes any portion of the test incorrectly, the trial is stopped, considered invalid, and restarted.
2. The test administrator begins timing on the "go" command and stops timing when the test performer backpedals through the line.
3. The best time is recorded as the final score.

Checklist: The test performer must

1. Understand how to run the course
2. Start with the body facing cone B

3. Turn *right* around cone B and *left* around cone C
4. Finish the test by backpedaling through the finish line
5. Actively recover between shuttles

Reference

Coaches roundtable: Testing for football. (1983). *National Strength and Conditioning Association Journal, 5*(5), 12–19.

■ 4-CORNER SHUTTLE RUN TEST

Objective: Measure running agility

Age Range: High school to college age

Equipment Needed:

1. Stopwatch
2. Tape measure
3. Four cones
4. Flat, open surface

Additional Personnel Needed: None

Setup:

1. The cones are used to create a square that is 7 yards (6.4 meters) long on each side (**Figure 10-14**).
2. The test performer may practice performing this test (described below) at partial speed.
3. The test performer stands behind cone A, facing cone B on the *outside* of the course.

Administration and Directions:

1. On the test administrator's "go" command, the test performer *sprints* from cone A to cone B (refer to Figure 10-14).
2. The test performer then *carioca—sprinting sideways by rotating hips and crossing feet in front of each other—facing away* from the course from cone B to cone C.
3. The test performer then *backpedals* from cone C to cone D.
4. The test performer then *carioca facing the course* from cone D to cone A.
5. The test performer should walk and stretch between trials.
6. Two trials are performed.

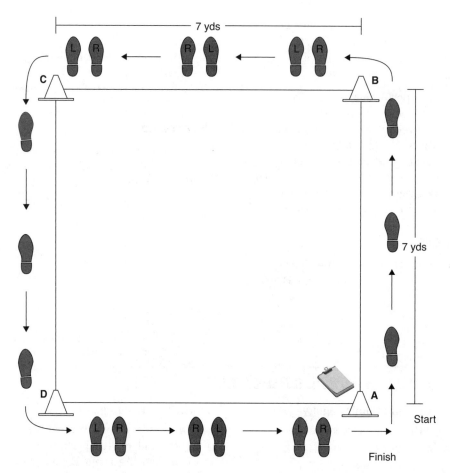

Figure 10-14 Four-Corner Shuttle Run Test Setup and Administration

Scoring:

1. If the test performer knocks over any cone or executes any portion of the test incorrectly, the trial is stopped, considered invalid, and restarted.
2. The test administrator begins timing on the "go" command and stops timing when the test performer carioca through cone A.
3. The best time is recorded as the final score.

Checklist: The test performer must

1. Understand how to run the course
2. Carioca in each direction
3. Perform this test slightly outside the cones
4. Actively recover between shuttles

Reference

Coaches roundtable: Testing for football. (1983). *National Strength and Conditioning Association Journal, 5*(5), 12–19.

■ BALSOM (SOCCER) AGILITY TEST

Objective: Measure running agility over a distance

Age Range: 10 to college age (originally designed for soccer athletes but can be utilized for similar athletes)

Equipment Needed:

1. Stopwatch
2. Tape measure
3. Ten cones
4. Soccer field (open grass field)

Additional Personnel Needed: One or two test assistants

Setup:

1. The course is 3 meters (3.2 yards) wide and 15 meters (16.4 yards) long with five 1-meter (1.1-yard)-wide gates (**Figure 10-15**).
2. The test administrator stands at the finish line, and a test assistant stands with the test performer at the starting line. An additional test assistant can be positioned inside the course to ensure the test performer complies with the test protocol.
3. The test performer may practice performing this test (described below) at partial speed.
4. The test performer starts inside gate A.

Administration and Directions:

1. On the test assistant's "go" command, the test performer *sprints* forward to gate B, touching the line with the foot (refer to Figure 10-15).
2. The test performer then stops and *sprints* back to gate A, touching the line with the foot.
3. The test performer then stops and *sprints* through gate C to gate D, touching the line with the foot.

4. The test performer then stops and *sprints* back to gate C, touching the line with the foot.
5. The test performer then stops and *sprints* through gate B and gate E.
6. One trial is performed.

Scoring:

1. If the test performer executes any portion of the test incorrectly, the trial is stopped, considered invalid, and restarted.
2. The test administrator starts timing when the test assistant gives the "go" command and stops timing when the test performer sprints through gate E.
3. The time is recorded as the final score.

Checklist: The test performer must

1. Understand how to run the course
2. Touch a cone or the space between each gate with a foot
3. Finish the test by sprinting through the final gate

References

Balsom, P. D. (1990). A field test to evaluate physical performance capacity of association football players. *Science and Football*, *3*, 9–11.

Ekblom, B. *Football (soccer)*. London: Blackwell Scientific Publications.

Sayers, A., Sayers, B. E., & Binkley H. (2008). Preseason fitness testing in National Collegiate Athletic Association soccer. *Strength and Conditioning Journal*, *30*(2), 70–75.

Svensson, M., & Drust, B. (2005). Testing soccer players. *Journal of Sports Sciences*, *23*(6), 601–618.

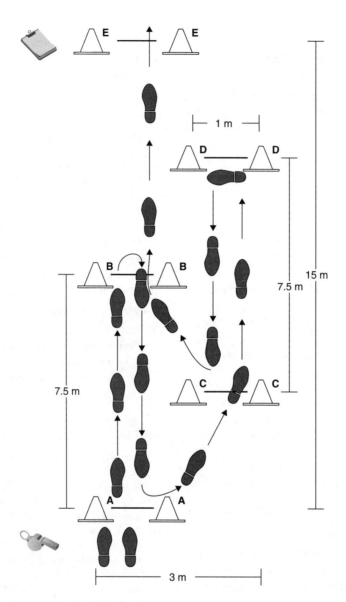

Figure 10-15 Balsom Agility Test Setup and Administration

■ HEXAGON TEST

Objective: Measure agility while jumping and balancing

Age Range: Middle school to college age

Equipment Needed:

1. Stopwatch
2. Tape measure
3. Floor tape
4. Large, flat floor area

Additional Personnel Needed: Test assistant

Setup:

1. The floor tape is used to create a hexagon with each side 2 feet (61 centimeters) long on the floor. Each angle of the hexagon should be 120°. An X may be created in the center of the hexagon. The X serves as a landing reference for the test performer (**Figure 10-16**).

2. The test performer may practice performing this test (described below) at partial speed.

3. The test performer begins in the center of the hexagon facing outward toward the test administrator. A test assistant may stand on the opposite side of the hexagon.

Administration and Directions:

1. On the test administrator's "go" command, the test performer jumps forward with both feet from the center of the hexagon over the line he or she is facing, lands on both feet, and jumps back to the center of the hexagon while facing the same direction (refer to Figure 10-16).

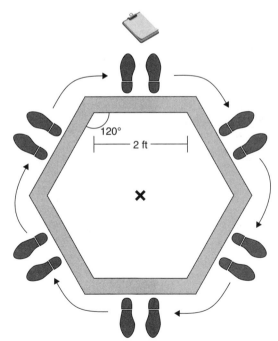

Figure 10-16   Hexagon Test Setup and Administration

2. The test performer continues to jump from the center of the hexagon over each line in a continuous *clockwise* motion until three complete revelations are performed, for a total of 18 jumps. The test performer faces the test administrator for the duration of this fitness test.

3. The test performer should end the test standing in the middle of the hexagon facing the test administrator.

4. The test performer should walk and stretch between trials.

5. Three trials are performed.

Scoring:

1. If the test performer executes any portion of the test incorrectly or significantly loses his or her balance, the trial is stopped, considered invalid, and restarted.

2. The test administrator begins timing on the "go" command and stops timing when the test performer has successfully completed all 18 jumps and is standing in the middle of the hexagon.

3. The best time is recorded as the final score.

Checklist: The test performer must

1. Have good balance and coordination before performing this test

2. Face outward at all times during this test

3. Jump over each line of the hexagon three times

4. Actively recover between trials

References

Baechle, T. R., & Earle, R. W. (2008). *Essentials of strength training and conditioning* (3rd ed.). Champaign, IL: Human Kinetics.

Farlinger, C. M., Kruisselbrink, L. D., & Fowles, J. R. (2007). Relationships to skating performance in competitive hockey players. *Journal of Strength and Conditioning Research, 21*(3), 915–922.

Pauole, K., Madole, K., Garhammer, J., Lacourse, M., & Rozenek, R. (2000). Reliability and validity of the T-test as a measure of agility, leg power, and leg speed in college-aged men and women. *Journal of Strength and Conditioning Research, 14*(4), 443–450.

Roetert, E. P., Brown, S. W., Piorkowski, P. A., & Woods, R. B. (1996). Fitness comparisons among three different levels of elite tennis players. *Journal of Strength and Conditioning Research, 10*(3), 139–143.

Roetert, E. P., Garrett, G. E., Brown, S. W., & Camaione, D. N. Performance profiles of nationally ranked junior tennis players. *Journal of Applied Sport Science Research, 6*(4), 225–231.

Roetert, E. P., Piorkowski, P. A., Woods, R. B., & Brown, S. W. (1995). Establishing percentiles for junior tennis players based on physical fitness testing results. *Clinics in Sports Medicine, 14*(1), 1–21.

■ 8-FEET UP-AND-GO TEST

Also Known as: Timed Up-and-Go Test

Objective: Measure agility in an elderly population; this test can also measure dynamic balance

Age Range: 60 to 90+

Equipment Needed:

1. Stopwatch
2. Tape measure
3. Straight back or folding chair with an approximate seat height of 17 inches (34 centimeters)
4. Cone
5. Wall
6. Flat floor at least 10 by 10 feet (3 by 3 meters)

Additional Personnel Needed: None

Setup:

1. The chair is placed against the wall (or otherwise secured to the floor), and the back of the cone is placed 8 feet (2.4 meters) directly in front of the chair (**Figure 10-17**).
2. The test performer may practice the test protocol (described below) at partial speed.

3. The test performer sits in the chair, with the hands on the thighs and feet flat on the floor.

Administration and Directions:

1. On the test administrator's "go" command, the test performer stands up from the chair (using the hands to push off is permitted) and *walks* around the cone (refer to Figure 10-17).
2. The test performer then returns to the seated position as quickly as possible after walking around the cone.
3. Two trials are performed.

Scoring:

1. If the test performer executes any portion of the test incorrectly, the trial is stopped, considered invalid, and restarted.
2. The test administrator begins timing on the "go" command and stops timing when the test performer returns to the starting position.
3. The best time is recorded as the final score.

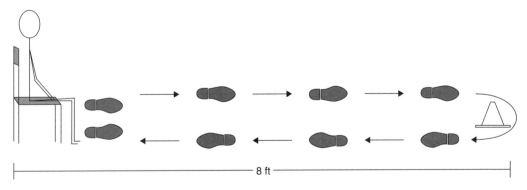

Figure 10-17   8-Feet Up-and-Go Test Setup and Administration

Checklist: The test performer must

1. Have good general balance and movement ability before performing this test
2. Begin from the proper seated position
3. Walk the course and not run

References

Cavani, V., Mier, C. M., Musto, A. A., & Tummers, N. (2002). Effects of a 6-week resistance-training program on functional fitness of older adults. *Journal of Aging and Physical Activity, 10,* 443–452.

Morrow, J. R., Jackson, A. W., Disch, J. G., & Mood, D. P. (2005). *Measurement and evaluation in human performance* (3rd ed.). Champaign, IL: Human Kinetics.

Podsiadlo, D., & Richardson, S. (1991). The timed "up & go": A test of basic functional mobility for frail elderly persons. *Journal of the American Geriatric Society, 39,* 142–148.

Rikli, R. E., & Jones, C. J. (1997). Assessing physical performance in independent older adults: Issues and guidelines. *Journal of Aging and Physical Activity, 5*(3), 244–261.

Rikli, R. E., & Jones, C. J. (1999). Development and validation of a functional fitness test for community-residing older adults. *Journal of Aging and Physical Activity, 7,* 129–161.

Rikli, R. E., & Jones, C. J. (1999). Functional fitness normative scores for community-residing older adults, ages 60–94. *Journal of Aging and Physical Activity, 7*(2), 162–181.

Rikli, R. E., & Jones, C. J. (2001). *Senior fitness test manual.* Champaign, IL: Human Kinetics.

CHAPTER

11

Speed, Speed Endurance, and Acceleration Testing

S peed, speed endurance, and acceleration are interrelated and affect each other. However, they can be tested separately if the test administrator understands how to isolate each component. All are tested linearly with proper timing and starting techniques. *Speed* is the movement per unit of time an individual runs a set distance and achieves maximum velocity. Speed tests are not generally performed for distances greater than 200 meters. *Speed endurance* is the ability to maintain maximum velocity during multiple repeated maximal accelerations and trials. Speed endurance is measured by performing maximum linear running trials (over a set distance) multiple times, indicating how well the test performer can maximally run over time. *Acceleration* is how rapidly a test performer can achieve maximum speed. Acceleration can be measured from a complete stop or from a partial movement (walk or jog).

To test for speed, speed endurance, and acceleration, the test administrator should ensure the test performer properly warms up and practices starting before any trials begin. The test performer should not be suffering any injury, particularly to the hamstrings, before any speed, speed-endurance, or acceleration tests are conducted. If a test performer experiences any tightness, soreness, or injury while performing any of these tests, the test should be stopped. During the test, the test performer should be instructed and encouraged to run through the finish line. If multiple trials are administered, the test performer should be encouraged to stretch and perform light physical activity between trials to clear as much lactic acid from the muscles as possible.

■ 40-YARD (37-METER) SPRINT (DASH) TEST

Objective: Measure linear sprinting speed and acceleration

Age Range: 10 to college age

Equipment Needed:

1. Stopwatch or an electronic timing system
2. Flat running surface with start and finish lines 40 yards (37 meters) apart, with at least 20 yards (18 meters) behind the finish line so that the test performer can decelerate safely

Additional Personnel Needed: Test assistant

Setup:

1. The test performer should practice starting prior to the test.
2. The test assistant lines up perpendicular to the starting line and is responsible for starting the test performer.
3. The test administrator lines up perpendicular to the finish line and is responsible for timing the trial.
4. The test performer lines up in either a 3- or 4-point stance behind the starting line (**Figure 11-1**).

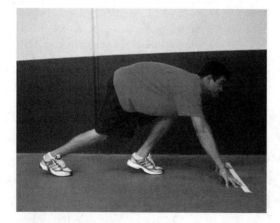

Figure 11-1 3-Point Stance

Administration and Directions:

1. On the test assistant's "go" command, the test performer maximally *sprints*, through the finish line.
2. The test performer should walk and stretch between trials.
3. Two trials are performed.

Scoring:

1. If an electronic timing system is utilized, a time will be given. The test administrator should confirm the electronic timing system is working during the trial.
2. If a stopwatch is utilized, it may be started either on the test performer's first movement or on the downward movement of the test assistant's arm. The timer should have a clear view of the finish line to stop timing when the test performer's chest crosses the finish line.
3. If hand timing is performed, it may be converted to an electronic time.
4. Each trial is timed to the nearest 0.1 seconds.
5. The best overall time is recorded as the final score.

Checklist: The test performer must

1. Have the entire body behind the starting line
2. Sprint maximally through the finish line
3. Actively recover between sprints

Note: This basic protocol can be utilized for distances up to 40 yards (37 meters). Distances of 5 to 20 yards (4.5 to 18 meters) measure acceleration.

References

American Association for Health, Physical Education, Recreation, and Dance (AAHPERD). (1976). *AAHPER youth fitness test manual.* Washington, DC: AAHPERD.

Baechle, T. R., & Earle, R. W. (2008). *Essentials of strength training and conditioning* (3rd ed.). Champaign, IL: Human Kinetics.

Baker, D., & Nance, S. (1999). The relation between running speed and measures of strength and power in professional rugby league players. *Journal of Strength and Conditioning Research, 13*(3), 230–235.

Brodie, D. A. (1996). *A reference manual for human performance measurement in the field of physical education and sports sciences.* Lewiston, NY: Edwin Mellen Press.

Coaches roundtable: Testing for football. (1983). *National Strength and Conditioning Association Journal, 5*(5), 12–19.

Davis, D. S., Barnette, B. J., Kiger, J. T., Mirasola, J. J., & Young, S. M. (2004). Physical characteristics that Predict functional performance in Division I college football players. *Journal of Strength and Conditioning Research, 18*(1), 115–120.

Gabbett, T. J., Kelly, J. N., & Sheppard, J. M. (2008). Speed, change of direction speed, and reactive agility of rugby league players. *Journal of Strength and Conditioning Research, 22*(1), 174–181.

Kuzmits, F. E., & Adams, A. J. The NFL Combine: Does it predict performance in the National Football League? *Journal of Strength and Conditioning Research, 22*(6), 1721–1727.

Mayhew, J. L., Bemben, M. G., Rohrs, D. M., & Bemben, D. A. (1994). Specificity among anaerobic power tests in college female athletes. *Journal of Strength and Conditioning Research, 8*(1), 43–47.

McGee, K. J., & Burkett, L. N. (2003). The National Football League Combine: A reliable predictor of draft status. *Journal of Strength and Conditioning Research, 17*(1), 6–11.

McSwegin, P., Pemberton, C., Petray, C., & Going, S. (1989). *Physical best: The AAHPERD guide to physical fitness education and assessment.* Reston, VA: AAHPERD.

Meir, R., Newton, R., Curtis, E., Fardell, M., & Butler, B. (2001). Physical fitness qualities of professional rugby league football players: Determination of positional differences. *Journal of Strength and Conditioning Research, 15*(4), 450–458.

Mirkov, D., Nedeljkovic, A., Kukolj, M., Ugarkovic, D., & Jaric, S. (2008). Evaluation of the reliability of soccer-specific field tests. *Journal of Strength and Conditioning Research, 22*(4), 1046–1050.

Moore, A. N., Decker, A. J., Baarts, J. N., DuPont, A. N., et al. (2007). Effect of competitiveness on forty-yard dash performance in college men and women. *Journal of Strength and Condition Research, 21*(2),385–388.

Murphy, A. J., & Wilson, G. J. (1997). The ability of tests of muscular function to reflect training-induced changes in performance. *Journal of Sports Sciences, 15*, 191–200.

Nesser, T. W., Huxel, K. C., Tincher, J. L., & Okada, T. (2008). The relationship between core stability and performance in division I football players. *Journal of Strength and Conditioning Research, 22*(6), 1750–1754.

Pauole, K., Madole, K., Garhammer, J., Lacourse, M., & Rozenek, R. (2000). Reliability and validity of the T-test as a measure of agility, leg power, and leg speed in college-aged men and women. *Journal of Strength and Conditioning Research, 14*(4), 443–450.

Safrit, M. J. (1995). *Complete guide to youth fitness testing.* Champaign, IL: Human Kinetics.

Sayers, A., Eveland-Sayers, B., & Binkley, B. (2008). Preseason fitness testing in National Collegiate Athletic Association soccer. *Strength and Conditioning Journal, 30*(4), 70–75.

Semenick, D. (1981). Conditioning program: Testing and evaluation. *National Strength and Conditioning Association Journal, 3*(2), 8–9.

Sierer, S. P., Battaglini, C. L., Mihalik, J. P., Shields, E. W., & Tomasini, N. T. (2008). The National Football League Combine: Performance differences between drafted and nondrafted players entering the 2004 and 2005 drafts. *Journal of Strength and Conditioning Research, 22*(1), 6–12.

Svensson, M., & Drust, B. (2005). Testing soccer players. *Journal of Sports Sciences, 23*(6), 601–618.

■ KALAMEN 50-YARD (45.5-METER) TEST

Also Known as: "Flying Start" Test

Objective: Measure linear speed endurance; a "flying start" test is considered more applicable to athletics and activity because many activities require the individual to go from partial to full speed rapidly

Age Range: Junior high to college age

Equipment Needed:

1. Stopwatch
2. Tape measure
3. 100-yard (91.4-meter) straight, flat surface
4. Three cones

Additional Personnel Needed: Test assistant

Setup:

1. One cone is placed at the starting line, one cone is placed 15 yards (13.7 meters) past the first cone, and one cone is placed 50 yards (45.7 meters) past the second cone (**Figure 11-2**).
2. The test administrator stands perpendicular to the finish line, and the test assistant stands perpendicular to cone B.

3. The test assistant is responsible for informing the test administrator when to begin timing the trial.
4. The test administrator stands perpendicular to the finish line and is responsible for timing the trial.
5. The test performer stands behind cone A, facing cone B.

Administration and Directions:

1. Once the test administrator signals he or she is ready to time the trial, the test performer begins running toward cone B. The test performer should slowly accelerate with the objective of being at full speed when cone B is reached (refer to Figure 11-2).
2. Once cone B is reached, the test performer *sprints* past cone C.
3. As the test performer passes cone B, the test assistant drops his or her arm, signaling the test administrator to begin timing the trial.
4. The test performer should walk and stretch between trials.

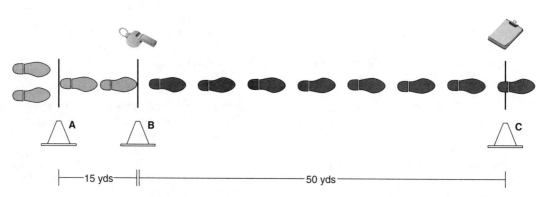

Figure 11-2   Kalamen 50-Yard Test Setup and Administration

5. Two trials are performed.

Scoring:

1. Each trial is timed and recorded.
2. The best overall time is recorded as the final score.

Checklist: The test performer must

1. Not begin to sprint from cone A
2. Be at a full sprint when he or she reaches cone B
3. Sprint past cone C
4. Actively recover between shuttles

Note: This basic test protocol can be used for other sprint and "flying start" distances.

References

Coaches roundtable: Testing for football. (1983). *National Strength and Conditioning Association Journal, 5*(5), 12–19.

Little, T., & Williams, A. G. (2005). Specificity of acceleration, maximum speed, and agility in professional soccer players. *Journal of Strength and Conditioning Research, 19*(1), 76–78.

Mirkov, D., Nedeljkovic, A., Kukolj, M., Ugarkovic, D., & Jaric, S. (2008). Evaluation of the reliability of soccer-specific field tests. *Journal of Strength and Conditioning Research, 22*(4), 1046–1050.

Sayers, A., Eveland Sayers, B., & Binkley, B. (2008). Preseason fitness testing in National Collegiate Athletic Association soccer. *Strength and Conditioning Journal, 30*(4), 70–75.

Semenick, D. (1984). Anaerobic testing: Practical applications. *National Strength and Conditioning Association Journal, 6*(5), 45, 70–73.

Svensson, M., & Drust, B. (2005). Testing soccer players. *Journal of Sports Sciences, 23*(6), 601–618.

■ 40-YARD (36.5-METER) REPEATED SPRINT TEST

Objective: Measure linear speed-endurance

Age Range: High school to college age

Equipment Needed:

1. Three stopwatches
2. Tape measure
3. Four cones
4. 100-yard (91.5-meter) straight, flat running surface

Additional Personnel Needed: Two test assistants

Setup:

1. The four cones are placed 20 yards (18.2 meters) apart in a straight line (**Figure 11-3**).

2. A test assistant stands perpendicular to line A, and the other test assistant stands perpendicular to line D.
3. The test administrator stands perpendicular to line C.
4. The test performer lines up behind line A, facing line C.

Administration and Directions:

1. On the test assistant's "go" command, the test performer *sprints* through line C (refer to Figure 11-3).
2. After passing line C, the test performer *decelerates* to line D.

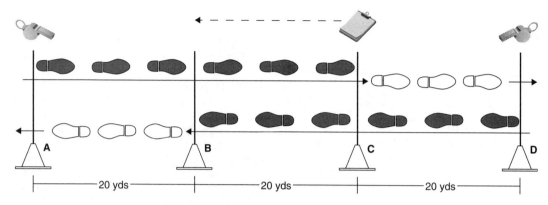

Figure 11-3   40-Yard Repeated Sprint Test Setup and Administration

3. The test performer is given 25 seconds to recover before the next sprint trial is performed.
4. The test performer should walk and stretch between sprints.
5. The test administrator moves from line C to line B.
6. The test assistant at line D signals the test performer to begin the next *sprint* from line D through line B.
7. This process continues until 10 sprints are performed.
8. One complete trial is performed.

Scoring:

1. Each sprint trial is timed and recorded.
2. The test performer's slowest sprint time is multiplied by 10.
3. The 10 sprint times are added together.
4. A percentile score is calculated.

> percentile score = [total sprint time ÷
>   (slowest sprint time × 10)]
>   × 100

5. The percentile score is recorded as the final score.

6. Any percentile score over 85% is considered "good."

Checklist: The test performer must

1. Sprint through each finish line
2. Understand he or she must be behind the next starting line and ready to sprint after the recovery period
3. Actively recover between sprints

Note: This basic protocol can be used for sprints of different distances. The rest period should be adjusted for sprints of different distances.

References

Coaches roundtable: Testing for football. (1983). *National Strength and Conditioning Association Journal, 5*(5), 12–19.

Semenick, D. (1984). Anaerobic testing: Practical applications. *National Strength and Conditioning Association Journal, 6*(5), 45, 70–73.

Svensson, M., & Drust, B. (2005). Testing soccer players. *Journal of Sports Sciences, 23*(6), 601–618.

■ BANGSBO SPRINT TEST

Also Known as: Repeated 34-Meter (37-Yard) Sprint Test

Objective: Measure linear speed endurance

Age Range: High school to college age

Equipment Needed:

1. Two stopwatches
2. Tape measure
3. Twelve posts at least 160 centimeters (63 inches) high *or* 12 cones
4. Open grass field

Additional Personnel Needed: Test assistant

Setup:

1. Six gates are created along a 40-meter (43.7-yard)-long course (**Figure 11-4**).
2. The test assistant stands perpendicular to gate A and is responsible for starting the test performer from gate A and keeping the active recovery time.

3. The test administrator stands perpendicular to gate B and is responsible for timing the test performer on the course.
4. The test performer lines up behind gate A, facing gate B.

Administration and Directions:

1. On the test assistant's "go" command, the test performer *sprints* from gate A through gate B" (refer to Figure 11-4).
2. After passing through gate B, the test performer slows down to a *jog*, goes through gate C, and *jogs* back to gate A.
3. The test performer has 25 seconds to actively recover after passing through gate B before the next sprinting trial begins.

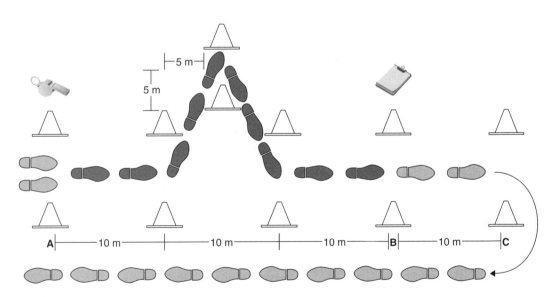

Figure 11-4   Bangsbo Sprint Test Setup and Administration

4. Seven sprints are completed (six recovery jogs).
5. One complete test is performed.

Scoring:

1. Each sprint trial is timed and recorded.
2. The final score is recorded as one of the following.
   a. The fastest single sprint time
   b. The mean time of the seven sprints

fatigue index = slowest sprint time of the last two sprints – fastest sprint time of the first two sprints

Checklist: The test performer must

1. Jog (without stopping or sitting down) during the 25-second active recovery period
2. Be back at gate A at the conclusion of the 25-second active recovery period
3. Go between all gates
4. Actively recover between sprints

References

Abrantes, C., Macas, V., & Sampaio, J. (2004). Variation in football players' sprint test performance across different ages and levels of competition. *Journal of Sports Science and Medicine, 3,* 44–49.

Ekblom, B. (1994). *Football (Soccer).* London: Blackwell Scientific Publications.

Sayers, A., Eveland Sayers, B., & Binkley, B. (2008). Preseason fitness testing in National Collegiate Athletic Association soccer. *Strength and Conditioning Journal, 30*(4), 70–75.

Svensson, M., & Drust, B. (2005). Testing soccer players. *Journal of Sports Sciences, 23*(6), 601–618.

Wragg, C. B., Maxwell, N. S., & Doust, J. H. (2000). Evaluation of the reliability and validity of a soccer-specific field test of repeated spring ability. *European Journal of Applied Physiology, 83,* 77–83.

■ 10-METER (10.9-YARD) TRIANGLE SPRINT TEST

Objective: Measure linear speed endurance

Age Range: High school to college age

Equipment Needed:

1. Stopwatch
2. Tape measure
3. Three cones
4. Lined soccer field; specifically, the penalty box

Additional Personnel Needed: Test assistant

Setup:

1. A 10-meter (10.9-yard) equilateral triangle is created on a lined soccer field adjacent to one corner of the penalty box. This is the sprint circuit (**Figure 11-5**).

2. The penalty box is utilized as the recovery circuit.
3. The test administrator and test assistant stand perpendicular to point A.
4. The test performer lines up on the sprint circuit behind point A, facing point B.

Administration and Directions:

1. On the test administrator's "go" command, the test performer *sprints* from point A to point B and from point B to point C, finishing back at point A (refer to Figure 11-5).
2. After finishing the sprint circuit, the test performer moves directly to the recovery circuit and *lightly jogs* the recovery circuit.

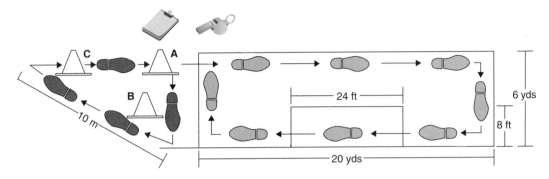

Figure 11-5   10-Meter Triangle Sprint Test Setup and Administration

3. The test performer has 42 seconds to complete the recovery circuit (active recovery) before the next sprint circuit is performed. The test performer should walk and lightly jog on the recovery circuit. The test assistant is responsible for monitoring the recovery time and ensuring the test performer completes the entire recovery circuit.

4. After 42 seconds have elapsed, the test performer should be back at point A of the sprint circuit and begin the next sprint circuit.

5. A total of 20 sprint circuits are completed (19 recovery circuits).

6. One complete trial is performed.

Scoring:

1. Each sprint trial is timed and recorded.

2. The final score is recorded as one of the following.

   a. The fastest single sprint time.

   b. The sum of the 20 sprint times.

   c. fatigue index = mean of the first two sprint times) – mean of the last two sprint times

Checklist: The test performer must

1. Jog (without stopping or sitting down) during the 42-second recovery circuit

2. Be back at gate A at the conclusion of the 42-second recovery circuit

3. Maximally sprint the sprint circuit

4. Actively recover on the recovery circuit, but not sit down

Reference

Ekblom, B. (1994). *Football (Soccer)*. London: Blackwell Scientific Publications.

Index

1-Leg Hop for Distance (OLHD) Test, 116–118
1-Leg Hop Test, 116–118
1-Mile or 1.5 Mile Run/Walk Test, 144–145
1-Repetition Maximum (1RM) Bench Press Test, 96–97
1-Repetition Maximum (1RM) Squat Test, 98–99
2-Minute Step-In-Place Test, 153–154
3-Cone Drill, 212–213
3-Corner Shuttle Run Test, 212–213
3-Hop Test, 118–119
3-Mile (4.8-Kilometer) Walk Test, 150
3-Minute Step Test, YMCA, 154–155
4-Corner Shuttle Run Test, 215–216
5-10-5 Test, 210–211
5-Jump Test, 120–121
5-Meter (5.5-Yard) Multiple Shuttle Test, 190–192
6-Minute Walking Test, 150–152
8-Feet Up-and-Go Test, 221–222
10-Meter (10.9-Yard) Triangle Sprint Test, 230–231
15-Meter Shuttle Test, 207–208
20-Meter Shuttle Run (20-MSR) Test, 167–169

20-Yard (22.8-Meter) Shuttle Test, 210–211
30-Second Chair Stand Test, 71–72
40-Meter Maximal Shuttle Run (40-M MST) Test, 185–186
40-Yard (36.5-Meter) Repeated Sprint Test, 227–228
40-Yard (37-Meter) Sprint (Dash) Test, 224–225
60-Yard (54.8-Meter) Shuttle Test, 178–179
300-Yard (272-Meter) Shuttle Test, 179–180
505 A–210

A
AAHPERD Shuttle Run Test, 200–202
Abdominal Curl for Endurance Test, 68–69
abdominal muscles
    power testing
        Standing Medicine Ball Throw Test, 137–138
    strength and endurance tests
        Abdominal Curl for Endurance Test, 68–69
        Abdominal Stage Test, 101–104
        Activitygram®, 3
        Fitnessgram®, 3

abdominal skinfold measurement site, 12

absolute flexibility, defined, 23

absolute strength. *See also* muscular strength

    1-Repetition Maximum (1RM) Bench Press Test, 97

    1-Repetition Maximum (1RM) Squat Test, 99

    defined, 93

acceleration

    40-Yard (37-Meter) Sprint (Dash) Test, 224–225

    NFL (American Football) Test Battery, 6

acceleration testing, overview, 223

ACL injury detection

    1-Leg Hop Test, 116–118

    Hop and Stop Test, 127–130

ACSM Fitness Test, 4

activities of daily living, test batteries for, 3

Activitygram®, 3, 22

aerobic capacity

    1-Mile (1.6-Kilometer) Walk Test, 147–148

    1-Mile or 1.5 Mile Run/Walk Test, 144–145

    2-Minute Step-In-Place Test, 153–154

    3-Mile (4.8-Kilometer) Walk Test, 150

    6-Minute Walking Test, 150–152

    ACSM Fitness Test, 4

    Activitygram®, 3

    Continuous Multistage Fitness (MFT) Test, 167–169

    Cooper Test, 142–144

    Fitnessgram®, 3

    Functional Fitness Test for Community-Residing Older Adults, 5–6

    Harvard Step Test, 157–158

    Harvard Step Test for Elementary School-Aged Males and Females, 162–164

    Harvard Step Test for Junior and Senior High and College Females, 161–162

    Harvard Step Test for Junior and Senior High Males, 158–161

    Hoosier Endurance Shuttle Run Test, 164–165

    overview, 141–142

    President's Challenge Fitness Test, 5

    Progressive Aerobic Cardiovascular Endurance Run (PACER) Test, 165–167

    Queens College Step Test, 155–156

    Rockport 1-Mile (1.6-Kilometer) Fitness Walking Test, 148–149

    Submaximal Mile (1.6-Kilometer) Track Jog Test, 146–147

    YMCA 3-Minute Step Test, 154–155

    YMCA Physical Fitness Test, 4

    Yo-Yo Endurance (Continuous) Test, 169–171

    Yo-Yo Intermittent Endurance (YYIE) Test, 171–173

    Yo-Yo Intermittent Recovery (YYIR) Test, 173–176

agility testing

    3-Cone Drill, 212–213

    4-Corner Shuttle Run Test, 215–216

    8-Feet Up-and-Go Test, 221–222

    505 Agility Test, 209–210

    AAHPERD Shuttle Run Test, 200–202

    Balsom (Soccer) Agility Test, 217–218

    Barrow Zigzag Run Test, 202–203

    Edgren Side Step Test, 197–198

    Functional Fitness Test for Community-Residing Older Adults, 5–6

    Hexagon Test, 219–220

    Illinois Agility Test, 205–207

    Nebraska Agility Run Test, 214–215

    overview, 193

    President's Challenge Fitness Test, 5

    Pro-Agility Test, 210–211

    Right Boomerang Run Test, 194–195

    SEMO Agility Test, 198–200

    Sidestepping Test, 196

    T-Test, 203–205

    Up and Back (UAB) Agility Test, 207–208

aging. *See* elderly

anaerobic capacity testing
    5-Meter (5.5-Yard) Multiple Shuttle Test, 190–192
    40-Meter Maximal Shuttle Run (40-M MST) Test, 185–186
    60-Yard (54.8-Meter) Shuttle Test, 178–179
    300-Yard (272-Meter) Shuttle Test, 179–180
    Line Drill Test, 180–182
    NFL (American Football) Test Battery, 6
    overview, 177
    Repeated 220-Yard (201-Meter) Sprint Test, 188–190
    Repeated Shuttle Sprint Ability (RSSA) Test, 186–188
    Triple 120-Meter (131-Yard) Shuttle Test, 183–184
anaerobic power. *See* anaerobic capacity testing; power testing
Arm-Curl Test, 63–64
arms. *See* upper-body power testing; upper-body strength and endurance
athletes. *See also* agility; muscular power; speed testing
    body fat equations, 22
    Kalamen 50-Yard (45.5-Meter) Test, 226–227
    NFL (American Football) Test Battery, 6
    Triple 120-Meter (131-Yard) Shuttle Test, 183–184
    Yo-Yo Intermittent Endurance (YYIE) Test, 171–173
    Yo-Yo Intermittent Recovery (YYIR) Test, 173–176

B

back
    Back Extensor Endurance Test, 73–74
    Back-Saver Sit-and-Reach Test, 32–33
    Back Scratch Test, 43–45
    Modified Back-Saver Sit-and-Reach Test, 34–35
    Modified Sit-and-Reach Test, 26–27
    Sit-and-Reach Test, 24–25
    Sit-and-Reach Wall Test, 29–30
    V-Sit-and-Reach Test, 30–31
    YMCA Sit-and-Reach Test, 28–29
Balance Beam Walk Test, 82–83
balance testing. *See also* agility
    dynamic balance
        8-Feet Up-and-Go Test, 221–222
        Balance Beam Walk Test, 82–83
        defined, 75
        Functional Fitness Test for Community-Residing Older Adults, 5–6
        Modified Bass Dynamic Balance Test, 87–88
        Modified Sideward Leap Test, 89–90
        Star Excursion Balance Test (SEBT), 90–91
        Tandem Walking Test, 84–85
        Timed 360° Turn Test, 85–86
    Hexagon Test, 219–220
    Hop and Stop Test, 127–130
    overview, 75
    static balance
        Bass Stick Test (Crosswise), 79–81
        Bass Stick Test (Lengthwise), 78–79
        defined, 75
        Modified Bass Dynamic Balance Test, 87–88
        Modified Sideward Leap Test, 89–90
        Stork Stand Test, 76–77
        Tandem Stance Test, 81–82
Balsom (Soccer) Agility Test, 217–218
Bangsbo Sprint Test, 229–230
Barrow Zigzag Run Test, 202–203
Bass Stick Test (Crosswise), 79–81
Bass Stick Test (Lengthwise), 78–79
bench press tests
    1-Repetition Maximum (1RM) Bench Press Test, 96–97
    NFL-225 Bench Press Test, 50–52
    YMCA Bench Press Test, 48–49
Bent Knee Push-Ups Test, 61–62
bias, timing, 1–2
biceps, skinfold measurement site, 14

body composition
  ACSM Fitness Test, 4
  Activitygram®, 3
  body mass index (BMI), 16–18
  equations summary, 22
  Fitnessgram®, 3
  Functional Fitness Test for Community-
    Residing Older Adults, 5–6
  overview of, 7–8
  skinfold measurement sites
    abdominal site, 12
    biceps site, 14
    calf site, 16
    midaxillary site, 10
    pectoral site, 8
    subscapular site, 9
    suprailiac site, 11
    thigh site, 15
    triceps site, 12–13
  test batteries, types of, 3
  waist-to-hip ratio (WHR), 19–21
  YMCA Physical Fitness Test, 4
body mass index (BMI), 16–18

C

calf skinfold measurement site, 16
calipers, skinfold measurement sites, 7–8
cardiorespiratory fitness
  1-Mile (1.6-Kilometer) Walk Test, 147–148
  1-Mile or 1.5 Mile Run/Walk Test, 144–145
  2-Minute Step-In-Place Test, 153–154
  3-Mile (4.8-Kilometer) Walk Test, 150
  6-Minute Walking Test, 150–152
  Continuous Multistage Fitness (MFT) Test,
    167–169
  Cooper Test, 142–144
  Harvard Step Test, 157–158
  Harvard Step Test for Elementary School-
    Aged Males and Females, 162–164
  Harvard Step Test for Junior and Senior
    High and College Females, 161–162
  Harvard Step Test for Junior and Senior
    High Males, 158–161

  Hoosier Endurance Shuttle Run Test,
    164–165
  overview, 141–142
  Progressive Aerobic Cardiovascular
    Endurance Run (PACER) Test, 165–167
  Queens College Step Test, 155–156
  Rockport 1-Mile (1.6-Kilometer) Fitness
    Walking Test, 148–149
  Submaximal Mile (1.6-Kilometer) Track Jog
    Test, 146–147
  test batteries, types of, 3
  YMCA 3-Minute Step Test, 154–155
  Yo-Yo Endurance (Continuous) Test,
    169–171
  Yo-Yo Intermittent Endurance (YYIE) Test,
    171–173
  Yo-Yo Intermittent Recovery (YYIR) Test,
    173–176
cardiovascular efficiency score (CES), 161–162
Chair Sit-and-Reach Test, 35–37
Chair Stand Test, 30-Second, 71–72
chest. *See* upper-body power testing; upper-
  body strength and endurance testing
chest/pectoral skinfold measurement site, 8
children, tests for. *See also* body composition
  Activitygram®, 3
  body fat equations, 22
  Fitnessgram®, 3
  President's Challenge Fitness Test, 5
  Progressive Aerobic Cardiovascular
    Endurance Run (PACER) Test, 165–167
Cone-Drill, 3 cones, 212–213
Continuous Multistage Fitness (MFT) Test,
  167–169
coordination. *See* agility
Corner Shuttle Run, 3-corner, 212–213
Corner Shuttle Run, 4-corner, 215–216
Crossover Hop Test, 121–122
Curl-Up Test, 68–69

D

Dips for Endurance Test, 57–59
Dips for Strength Test, 106–107

dynamic balance. *See also* balance testing
   Balance Beam Walk Test, 82–83
   defined, 75
   Functional Fitness Test for Community-
      Residing Older Adults, 5–6
   Modified Bass Dynamic Balance Test, 87–88
   Modified Sideward Leap Test, 89–90
   Star Excursion Balance Test (SEBT), 90–91
   Tandem Walking Test, 84–85
   Timed 360° Turn Test, 85–86
Dynamometer Test, 94–95

E
Edgren Side Step Test, 197–198
elderly
   2-Minute Step-In-Place Test, 153–154
   8-Feet Up-and-Go, 221–222
   30-Second Chair Stand Test, 71–72
   Arm-Curl Test, 63–64
   Chair Sit-and-Reach Test, 35–37
   Functional Fitness Test for Community-
      Residing Older Adults, 5–6
   Timed 360° Turn Test, 85–86
electronic timing systems, 2
endurance. *See also* cardiorespiratory fitness;
   muscular endurance testing
   speed
      10-Meter (10.9-Yard) Triangle Sprint Test,
         230–231
      40-Yard (36.5-Meter) Repeated Sprint
         Test, 227–228
      Bangsbo Sprint Test, 229–230
      Kalamen 50-Yard (45.5-Meter) Test,
         226–227
      overview, 223
equations
   body mass index (BMI), 17
   cardiovascular efficiency score, 161–162
   distance traveled, 5-Meter (5.5-Yard)
      Multiple Shuttle Test, 191
   fatigue index
   40-Meter Maximal Shuttle Run (40-M MST)
      Test, 185–186

Repeated Shuttle Sprint Ability (RSSA) Test,
   186–188
   Shuttle Test, 191
   Sprint Test, 230
fitness index, 161–162
Hop and Stop Test, 127–130
percentage fatigue, 186, 187
percentile score, repeated sprints, 228
physical efficiency index (PEI), 157–158,
   160
relative strength
   1-Repetition Maximum (1RM) Bench
      Press, 97
   Dips for Strength Test, 107
   Pull-Ups for Strength Test, 105
Sargent's Test, 112
Side Hop Test, 127
Square Hop Test, 125
Submaximal Mile (1.6 kilometer) Track Jog
   Test, 147
Vane-Slat Apparatus Method, 115
VO_{2max} conversion
   1-Mile (1.6-Kilometer) Walk Test, 148
   1-Mile or 1.5 Mile Run/Walk Test, 144–
      145
   Continuous Multistage Fitness (MFT)
      Test, 168
   Cooper Test, 143
   Progressive Aerobic Cardiovascular
      Endurance Run (PACER) Test, 166–167
   Queens College Step Test, 156
   Rockport 1-Mile (1.6-Kilometer) Fitness
      Walking Test, 149
   Yo-Yo Intermittent Recovery (YYIR)
      Test, 175
equations for skinfold measurements, 8
equilibrium. *See* balance testing

F
fatigue index/percent, 5-Meter (5.5-Yard)
   Multiple Shuttle Test, 191
fatigue index, Repeated 34-Meter (37-Yard)
   Sprint Test, 230

fatigue index, 40-Meter Maximal Shuttle Run (40-M MST) Test, 185–186

fatigue index, Repeated Shuttle Sprint Ability (RSSA) Test, 186–188

females. *See also* body composition
  body fat equations, 22
  Harvard Step Test for Junior and Senior High and College Females, 161–162
  Modified Push-Ups for Endurance Test, 61–62
  Queens College Step Test, 156
  Submaximal Mile (1.6-Kilometer) Track Jog Test, 147

Fitnessgram®, 3, 22

fitness test batteries, overview, 2–3

Flexed Arm-Hang Test, 56–57

flexibility testing
  ACSM Fitness Test, 4
  Activitygram®, 3
  Back-Saver Sit-and-Reach Test, 32–33
  Back Scratch Test, 43–45
  Chair Sit-and-Reach Test, 35–37
  Fitnessgram®, 3
  Functional Fitness Test for Community-Residing Older Adults, 5–6
  Modified Back-Saver Sit-and-Reach Test, 34–35
  Modified Sit-and-Reach Test, 26–27
  overview, 23
  President's Challenge Fitness Test, 5
  Shoulder-and-Wrist Elevation Test, 42–43
  Shoulder Lift Test, 40–41
  Sit-and-Reach Test, 24–25
  Sit-and-Reach Wall Test, 29–30
  test batteries, types of, 3
  Trunk-and-Neck Extension Test, 39–40
  Trunk Lift Test, 37–38
  V-Sit-and-Reach Test, 30–31
  YMCA Physical Fitness Test, 4
  YMCA Sit-and-Reach Test, 28–29

Flying Start Test, 226–227

football athletes, tests for, 6

four-directional agility, 203–205

Functional Fitness Test for Community-Residing Older Adults, 5–6

G

general fitness test batteries
  ACSM Fitness Test, 4
  Fitnessgram®, 3
  President's Challenge Fitness Test, 5
  YMCA Physical Fitness Test, 4

H

hamstring muscles, flexibility
  Back-Saver Sit-and-Reach Test, 32–33
  Chair Sit-and-Reach Test, 35–37
  Modified Back-Saver Sit-and-Reach Test, 34–35
  Sit-and-Reach Test, 24–25
  Sit-and-Reach Test, modified, 26–27
  Sit-and-Reach Wall Test, 29–30
  V-Sit-and-Reach Test, 30–31
  YMCA Sit-and-Reach Test, 28–29

Handgrip Strength Test, 94–95

hand timing, conversion formula, 2

Harvard Step Test, 157–158

Harvard Step Test for Elementary School-Aged Males and Females, 162–164

Harvard Step Test for Junior and Senior High and College Females, 161–162

Harvard Step Test for Junior and Senior High Males, 158–161

health-related test batteries, overview, 3

height, conversion to meters, 17

Hexagon Test, 219–220

hips
  Sit-and-Reach Test, 24–25
  Sit-and-Reach Test, modified, 26–27
  Waist-to-Hip Ratio (WHR), 19–21

Hoosier Endurance Shuttle Run Test, 164–165

Hop, Stop, and Leap Test, 127–130

Hop and Stop Test, 127–130

Hop for Distance, 1-Leg (OLHD) Test, 116–118

Hop Test, 1-Leg, 116–118
Hop Test, 3-hop, 118–119

I
Illinois Agility Test, 205–207
injury detection
    1-Leg Hop Test, 116–118
    Hop and Stop Test, 127–130

J
joints. *See* flexibility
jump agility, Hexagon Test, 219–220
Jump Test, 5 jumps, 120–121

K
Kalamen 50-Yard (45.5-Meter) Test, 226–227
kilograms, conversion to, 17
knee injuries
    1-Leg Hop Test, 116–118
    Hop and Stop Test, 127–130

L
L-Drill/L-Run, 212–213
lateral agility
    Edgren Side Step Test, 197–198
    Sidestepping Test, 196
legs. *See* lower-body power testing; lower-body
  strength and endurance testing
Line Drill Test, 180–182
lower-body power testing
    1-Leg Hop Test, 116–118
    3-Hop Test, 118–119
    5-Jump Test, 120–121
    6-Meter Timed Hop Test, 123–124
    Backward Overhead Medicine Ball Throw
      Test, 139–140
    Crossover Hop Test, 121–122
    Hop and Stop Test, 127–130
    Sargent's Test, 112–113
    Side Hop Test, 126–127
    Square Hop Test, 124–125
    Standing Broad Jump Test, 110–111
    Vane-Slat Apparatus Method, 114–116

lower-body strength and endurance testing
    1-Repetition Maximum (1RM) Squat Test,
      98–99
    30-Second Chair Stand Test, 71–72
    Static Leg Endurance Test, 69–71

M
males. *See also* body composition
    body fat equations, 22
    Harvard Step Test for Junior and Senior
      High Males, 158–161
    Queens College Step Test, 156
    Submaximal Mile (1.6-Kilometer) Track Jog
      Test, 147
metric units, conversion to, 17
midaxillary skinfold measurement site, 10
mobility, Functional Fitness Test for
  Community-Residing Older Adults, 5–6
Modified Back-Saver Sit-and-Reach Test,
  34–35
Modified Bass Dynamic Balance Test, 87–88
Modified Pull-Ups for Endurance Test, 54–55
Modified Push-ups for Endurance Test, 61–62
Modified Sideward Leap Test, 89–90
Modified Sit-and-Reach Test, 26–27
Multiple Shuttle Test, 5-Meter (5.5-Yard),
  190–192
muscular endurance testing. *See also* muscular
  strength testing
    30-Second Chair Stand Test, 71–72
    Abdominal Curl for Endurance Test, 68–69
    ACSM Fitness Test, 4
    Arm-Curl Test, 63–64
    Back Extensor Endurance Test, 73–74
    Dips for Endurance Test, 57–59
    Flexed Arm-Hang Test, 56–57
    Functional Fitness Test for Community-
      Residing Older Adults, 5–6
    NFL-225 Bench Press Test, 50–52
    NFL (American Football) Test Battery, 6
    overview, 47
    President's Challenge Fitness Test, 5
    Pull-Ups for Endurance Test, 52–54

muscular endurance testing *(Continued)*
  Pull-Ups for Endurance Test, Modified, 54–55
  Push-Ups for Endurance Test, 59–61
  Push-Ups for Endurance Test, Modified, 61–62
  Sit-Ups for Endurance Test, 65–67
  Static Leg Endurance Test, 69–71
  test batteries, types of, 3
  YMCA Bench Press Test, 48–49
  YMCA Physical Fitness Test, 4
muscular power testing
  1-Leg Hop Test, 116–118
  3-Hop Test, 118–119
  5-Jump Test, 120–121
  6-Meter Timed Hop Test, 123–124
  Backward Overhead Medicine Ball Throw Test, 139–140
  Crossover Hop Test, 121–122
  Hop and Stop Test, 127–130
  NFL (American Football) Test Battery, 6
  overview, 109
  Sargent's Test, 112–113
  Seated Medicine Ball Throw Test, 131–132
  Seated Shot Put Test, 133–134
  Side Hop Test, 126–127
  Square Hop Test, 124–125
  Standing Broad Jump Test, 110–111
  Standing Medicine Ball Chest Pass Test, 135–136
  Standing Medicine Ball Throw Test, 137–138
  Vane-Slat Apparatus Method, 114–116
muscular strength testing. *See also* muscular endurance
  1-Repetition Maximum (1RM) Bench Press Test, 96–97
  1-Repetition Maximum (1RM) Squat Test, 98–99
  Abdominal Stage Test, 101–104
  Dips for Strength Test, 106–107
  Functional Fitness Test for Community-Residing Older Adults, 5–6

Handgrip Strength (Dynamometer) Test, 94–95
  overview, 93–94
  President's Challenge Fitness Test, 5
  Pull-Ups for Strength Test, 104–106
  Sit-Ups for Strength Test, 100–101
  test batteries, types of, 3
  YMCA Physical Fitness Test, 4

N
Nebraska Agility Run Test, 214–215
NFL-225 Bench Press Test, 50–52
NFL (American Football) Test Battery, 6

O
obesity/overweight
  body mass index (BMI), 16–18

P
pectoral skinfold measurement site, 8
Phantom Chair Test, 69–71
physical activities, test batteries types, 3
physical efficiency index (PEI), 157–158, 160
power testing
  1-Leg Hop Test, 116–118
  3-Hop Test, 118–119
  5-Jump Test, 120–121
  6-Meter Timed Hop Test, 123–124
  Backward Overhead Medicine Ball Throw Test, 139–140
  Crossover Hop Test, 121–122
  Hop and Stop Test, 127–130
  overview, 109
  Sargent's Test, 112–113
  Seated Medicine Ball Throw Test, 131–132
  Seated Shot Put Test, 133–134
  Side Hop Test, 126–127
  Square Hop Test, 124–125
  Standing Broad Jump Test, 110–111
  Standing Medicine Ball Chest Pass Test, 135–136

Standing Medicine Ball Throw Test, 137–138

Vane-Slat Apparatus Method, 114–116

President's Challenge Fitness Test, 5

Pro-Agility Test, 210–211

Progressive Aerobic Cardiovascular Endurance Run (PACER) Test, 165–167

Pull-Ups for Endurance Test, 52–54

Pull-Ups for Endurance Test, Modified, 54–55

Pull-Ups for Strength Test, 104–106

Push-ups for Endurance Test, 59–61

Push-ups for Endurance Test, Modified, 61–62

Q

Queens College Step Test, 155–156

R

range of motion. *See* flexibility

reaction-time delays, 2

relative flexibility, defined, 23

relative strength. *See also* muscular strength

    1-Repetition Maximum (1RM) Bench Press Test, 97

    1-Repetition Maximum (1RM) Squat Test, 99

    Dips for Strength Test, 107

    Pull-Ups for Strength Test, 105

relative strength, defined, 93

Repeated 34-Meter (37-Yard) Sprint Test, 229–230

Repeated 220-Yard (201-Meter) Sprint Test, 188–190

Repeated Shuttle Sprint Ability (RSSA) Test, 186–188

Repeated Sprint Ability (RSA) Test, 186–188

Repeated Sprint Test, 40-Yard (36.5-Meter), 227–228

Right Boomerang Run Test, 194–195

Rockport 1-Mile (1.6-Kilometer) Fitness Walking Test, 148–149

running agility

    3-Cone Drill, 212–213

    4-Corner Shuttle Run Test, 215–216

    505 Agility Test, 209–210

    AAHPERD Shuttle Run Test, 200–202

    Balsom (Soccer) Agility Test, 217–218

    Barrow Zigzag Run Test, 202–203

    Illinois Agility Test, 205–207

    Nebraska Agility Run Test, 214–215

    Pro-Agility Test, 210–211

    Right Boomerang Run Test, 194–195

    SEMO Agility Test, 198–200

    T-Test, 203–205

    Up and Back (UAB) Agility Test, 207–208

Running Repeated Sprint Ability (rRSA) Test, 186–188

running tests. See agility tests; cardiorespiratory fitness; shuttle tests; speed testing

run/walk tests

    1-Mile or 1.5 Mile Run/Walk Test, 144–145

    Cooper Test, 142–144

S

Sargent's Test, 112–113

Seated Medicine Ball Throw Test, 131–132

Seated Shot Put Test, 133–134

SEMO Agility Test, 198–200

senior citizens. See elderly

shoulder. See upper-body power testing; upper-body strength and endurance testing

Shoulder-and-Wrist Elevation Test, 42–43

Shoulder Lift Test, 40–41

Shoulder Stretch Test, 43–45

shuttle tests

    3-Cone Drill, 212–213

    4-Corner Shuttle Run Test, 215–216

    5-Meter (5.5-Yard) Multiple Shuttle Test, 190–192

    15-Meter Shuttle Test, 207–208

    20-Meter Shuttle Run (20-MSR) Test, 167–169

    20-Yard (22.8-Meter) Shuttle Test, 210–211

shuttle tests *(Continued)*
  40-Meter Maximal Shuttle Run (40-M MST)
    Test, 185–186
  60-Yard (54.8-Meter) Shuttle Test, 178–179
  300-Yard (272-Meter) Shuttle Test, 179–180
  Pro-Agility Test, 210–211
  Repeated Shuttle Sprint Ability (RSSA)
    Test, 186–188
  Triple 120-Meter (131-Yard) Shuttle Test,
    183–184
  Up and Back (UAB) Agility Test, 207–208
Side Hop Test, 126–127
Sidestepping Test, 196
Sit-and-Reach Test, 24–25
Sit-and-Reach Test (Modified), 26–27
Sit-and-Reach Wall Test, 29–30
Sit-Ups for Endurance Test, 65–67
Sit-Ups for Strength Test, 100–101
skill-related test batteries, overview, 3
skinfold measurement sites
  abdominal site, 12
  biceps site, 14
  calf site, 16
  midaxillary site, 10
  overview, 7–8
  pectoral site, 8
  subscapular site, 9
  suprailiac site, 11
  thigh site, 15
  triceps site, 12–13
Soccer Agility Test, 217–218
speed testing
  10-Meter (10.9-Yard) Triangle Sprint Test,
    230–231
  40-Yard (36.5-Meter) Repeated Sprint Test,
    227–228
  40-Yard (37-Meter) Sprint (Dash) Test,
    224–225
  60-Yard (54.8-Meter) Shuttle Test, 178–179
  Bangsbo Sprint Test, 229–230
  Kalamen 50-Yard (45.5-Meter) Test, 226–227
  NFL (American Football) Test Battery, 6
  overview, 223

Square Hop Test, 124–125
Squat Test, 1-Repetition Maximum (1RM),
  98–99
Standing Broad Jump Test, 110–111
Standing Medicine Ball Throw Test, 137–138
Star Excursion Balance Test (SEBT), 90–91
static balance. *See also* balance testing
  Bass Stick Test (Crosswise), 79–81
  Bass Stick Test (Lengthwise), 78–79
  defined, 75
  Stork Stand Test, 76–77
  Tandem Stance Test, 81–82
Static Leg Endurance Test, 69–71
Step-In-Place Test, 2-Minute, 153–154
Step Test, YMCA, 154–155
stopwatch, guidelines for use, 1–2
Stork Stand Test, 76–77
strength testing. *See* muscular strength
Submaximal Mile (1.6 kilometer) Track Jog
  Test, 146–147
subscapular skinfold measurement site, 9
Suicide Test/Drill, 180–182
suprailiac skinfold measurement site, 11

T
Tandem Stance Test, 81–82
Tandem Walking Test, 84–85
test batteries, overview, 2–3
thigh. *See also* lower-body power testing;
  lower-body strength and endurance testing
    muscle endurance tests, 69–71
    skinfold measurement site, 15
Timed 360° Turn Test, 85–86
timing, guidelines for, 1–2
Triangle Sprint Test, 10-Meter (10.9-Yards),
  230–231
triceps skinfold measurement site, 12–13
Triple 120-Meter (131-Yard) Shuttle Test,
  183–184
Triple-Hop (Jump) Test, 118–119
trunk
  Activitygram®, 3
  Fitnessgram®, 3

flexibility, 37–40
Trunk-and-Neck Extension Test, 39–40
Trunk Flexion Test, 24–25
Trunk Lift Test, 37–38
T-Test, 203–205
Turn Test, Timed 360°, 85–86

U
underweight, body mass index (BMI),
  16–18
Up and Back (UAB) Ability Test, 207–208
upper-body power testing
  Backward Overhead Medicine Ball
    Throw Test, 139–140
  Seated Medicine Ball Throw Test,
    131–132
  Standing Medicine Ball Chest Pass Test,
    135–136
  Standing Medicine Ball Throw Test,
    137–138
upper-body strength and endurance
 testing
  1-Repetition Maximum (1RM) Bench Press
    Test, 96–97
  Activitygram®, 3
  Arm Curl Test, 63–64
  Dips for Endurance Test, 57–59
  Dips for Strength Test, 106–107
  Fitnessgram®, 3
  Flexed Arm Hang, 56–57
  NFL-225 Bench Press Test, 50–52
  Pull-Ups for Endurance Test, 52–54
  Pull-Ups for Endurance Test, Modified,
    54–55
  Pull-Ups for Strength Test, 104–106
  Push-Ups for Endurance Test, 59–61
  YMCA Bench Press Test, 48–49

V
Valsalva maneuver, 93–94
Vane-Slat Apparatus Method, 114–116
Vertical Jump Test, 114–116
Vertical Jump Test: Wall Method, 112–113
V-Sit-and-Reach Test, 30–31

W
waist-to-hip ratio (WHR), 19–21
walking agility, 8-Feet Up-and-Go Test, 221–222
walking tests
  1-Mile (1.6-Kilometer) Walk Test, 147–148
  3-Mile (4.8-Kilometer) Walk Test, 150
  6-Minute Walking Test, 150–152
  Balance Beam Walk Test, 82–83
  Rockport 1-Mile (1.6-Kilometer) Fitness
    Walking Test, 148–149
  Tandem Walking Test, 84–85
walk/run tests
  1-Mile or 1.5 Mile Run/Walk Test, 144–145
  Cooper Test, 142–144
Wall Sit Test, 69–71
weight, conversion to kilograms, 17
women. *See* females
wrist, flexibility, 42–43

Y
YMCA 3-Minute Step Test, 154–155
YMCA Bench Press Test, 48–49
YMCA Half Sit-Up Test, 68–69
YMCA Physical Fitness Test, 4, 22
YMCA Sit-and-Reach Test, 28–29
Yo-Yo Endurance (Continuous) Test, 169–171
Yo-Yo Intermittent Endurance (YYIE) Test,
  171–173
Yo-Yo Intermittent Recovery (YYIR) Test,
  173–176